PRIMARY HEALTH CARE

PRIMARY HEALTH CARE

Medicine in its place

John J. Macdonald

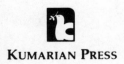

KUMARIAN PRESS

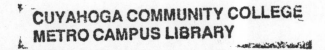

Published in the United States of America by Kumarian Press, Inc.
630 Oakwood Avenue, Suite 119, West Hartford, Connecticut
06110-1529 USA
ISBN 1-56549-024-X (U.S.)

Published in the United Kingdom by Earthscan Publications Ltd.
120 Pentonville Road, London N1 9JN United Kingdom
ISBN 1-85383-112-3 (U.K.)

Printed and bound in Great Britain by Biddles Ltd.,
Guildford and King's Lynn.
First Printed in 1993

Cover design by Zoe Davenport
Typeset by DP Photosetting, Aylesbury, Bucks

Library of Congress Cataloging-in-Publication Data

Macdonald, John J., 1943.
        Primary health care: medicine in its place
                p.   cm.—(Kumarian press library of management for
        development)
        Includes bibliographical references and index.
        ISBN 1-56549-024-X (pbk.)
        1. Primary health care. I. Title. II. Series.
        [DNLM: 1. Primary Health Care. W 84.6 M135p 1993]
        RA427 .9 .M33   1993
        362.1'0425   92-46103

97   96   95   94   93   5   4   3   2   1

Contents

Acknowledgements

The book owes much to other people. When I was a practitioner of PHC in Africa, coordinating a village-based health and development programme, I owed much to the people of the part of Zambia where I worked. Their spirit of resilience in the face of often difficult circumstances changed my life and enriched it considerably. Without the friendship of such village health workers as Clement Sebente and professional midwives such as Eva Nillson and the late Christina Nkole I could have achieved very little. The doctors and nurses I worked with influenced me, notably Bobby Hultberg, Beaudouin Peters and Murielle Koks-Bosch and I was supported in much of the work I tried to initiate by Dr. Raf Carmen, to whose friendship in those days I owe much. Dr. Mary Lyon in Sierra Leone, Dr. Samir Chaudri of the Child in Need Institute in India and Professor Banerji in Delhi are towering figures whose example has kept me believing in PHC. Since my days in Africa I have been privileged to work with health workers from many countries who have followed courses in PHC run by me both in their countries and in Europe. I have tried to run participatory courses, building on the experiences and insights of participants, in the way PHC promotes and in the manner I learned in Africa. I hope the participants learned from me; I certainly have from them. Most of them I met when they were looking for new approaches to health care, aware of the need for change. Many, now back in the field, struggle to put the ideas of PHC into practice. In Europe I have been inspired by the work of people in communities who tackle the causes of ill-health as well as seeking help with its symptoms, such as Cathy McCormack and her colleagues in the Easterhall Tenants' Association in Glasgow in their struggle for healthier housing, as well as by Community Health Workers such as Jane Jones in Edinburgh who read and made helpful comments on this book. Mike Beveredige, David Johnson and Bernard Schlecht have offered the professional and moral support needed to write the book. With admiration, gratitude and affection, I dedicate this book to all of these and their struggle, as well as to my wife, Josna, my bonny son, Rohan, and the memory of my mother, Sarah Macdonald.

Introduction

This book is about Primary Health Care (PHC). The approach is well known and the subject of considerable debate in countries of the Third World where it has become incorporated into many national health programmes; it is less well known in industrialised countries. Almost everywhere it tends to be confused with primary *medical* care. In an international context, 'Primary Health Care' means an approach to the provision of health services which emphasises the *promotion* of health through a partnership between health and other professionals and the community, as well as a system of treatment and curative care based on meeting the health needs of the majority of the population to be served.

In most societies health care provision focuses mainly on curative care based in institutions and is mainly in the hands of the medical profession whose business it is. PHC presents us with the guidelines for a new approach to conceptualising and planning health care. New directions are certainly needed. The health care systems in most countries are undergoing difficult times, and serious questions are being asked about their effectiveness and their appropriateness. Everywhere health care is becoming more expensive and if only for this reason voices are being raised, at least from outside the medical profession, demanding that medical systems be subject to critical analysis. As we move towards the twenty-first century, it is a good time to ask: are we right to continue to develop our health care systems along the lines we have been following? In Western societies the current debate often has to do with the relative advantages and disadvantages of state and private provision and the decisions to be made about what diseases and conditions are priority for treatment and care. In the Third World situation, debate on what health care is best health care might seem like a luxury since many countries are struggling to maintain the standards which they set themselves at the time of independence, running just to keep standing still, as it were. Some would say that a debate such as this book would like to encourage is a luxury we cannot afford. I would say that the debate is a something we cannot afford to miss. The central issue of this debate is the one raised by the proponents of the Primary Health Care approach and might be expressed in this way: instead of 'more of the same', expanding the model of health care which we have now, do we not need a completely new kind of health care system? The PHC approach points the way towards such a new system.

The blueprint for a new health care system was laid out at the International Conference of Alma Ata in 1978, convened by WHO and UNICEF. The impetus for the conference came from concern about the health needs of countries of the Third World. It exposed problems of the existing health care systems in these countries, systems largely modelled on western health care, but failing to meet the basic health needs of many populations. The conference declared the need for change that many practitioners of health had felt for several decades; it also laid down the guidelines for a new way of thinking about and planning for health systems: the Primary Health Care approach. A development of the principles of this approach and some of its consequences for health systems and professionals form the core of this book.

The vocabulary of Alma Ata, of PHC, has become common currency in countries of Africa, Latin America and Asia. Debate is widespread in these countries concerning the need for further clarification of the principles of the approach and modes of application. In the West there seems to be little awareness or concern for these principles. Indeed, research in the 1980s showed that those responsible for public health training of doctors in Europe knew little of Alma Ata (Walton, 1983, 1985). One could perhaps describe this situation of the western medical reaction to Alma Ata as one, not of deafening silence, but of deafness.

Yet PHC might well be the Trojan horse of medical practice. In Greek legend, the people of Troy admitted within their walls a wooden horse because they found it harmless, even amusing. Yet it brought about their downfall because while they slept some of their enemies, the Greeks, emerged from inside the horse and opened the gates to the invading army. I would like to think of PHC as such an unexpected power for change. Its principles have been accepted on to the stage of international health care, perhaps because, since their focus was 'over there', in countries with little political, economic or medical influence on the world stage, it was assumed that they could have little relevance for western societies. No could they pose any threat to established ways of thinking and acting in the health profession in the West. Or at least, so it was thought. Such an attitude may come to be seen as the result of a gross underestimation of the force of the case for PHC.

The 'why' of PHC, the reasons for its emergence on the international stage as a health care strategy, is addressed in Chapter One of the book which looks at the failure of the conventional medical model to meet the health needs of many communities throughout the world. Chapter Two explains at greater length what is the nature of this medical model: if PHC is in any sense an alternative approach, it is necessary to see more clearly the medical framework for thought and action against which it is, in some sense, a reaction. The broad outlines of the PHC approach, the 'what' of PHC, are laid out in Chapter Three, and the rest of the book is in a sense a further elaboration of these outlines. There is an attempt to clarify further the principles of the approach as set out in Alma Ata and as yet insufficiently understood worldwide. Such a clarification may serve to show that there are individuals and groups working on new approaches to health care in western societies whose activities and aims are very recognisable in the context of PHC and in that sense are part of the international PHC movement. The rapid emergence of 'selective' versions of PHC in so-called developing countries after the Conference of Alma Ata and their popularity both with the medical profession and the medical aid agencies merit them a chapter on their own (Chapter Four). In many ways selective PHC can be seen as a refusal of the medical world to accept the challenge of comprehensive PHC and to incorporate it into existing ways of thinking and doing.

There are three 'pillars' of the PHC approach and they are developed at some length in this book. Once they have been accepted as having relevance for the health systems of the so-called developing countries it becomes legitimate, even necessary, to ask if they do not have relevance also for the health systems of the West, the source of the developing countries' health care model. Chapter Five develops the *participation* pillar of PHC, Chapter Six deals with the *intersectoral collaboration* pillar and Chapter Seven the *equity* pillar. I would suggest that these three 'essential elements' or pillars of PHC pose an enormous challenge to any health practitioner and any health system. This challenge is perhaps especially important in western societies where there seems to be little critical self-awareness on the part of members of the health profession, and a notable reluctance to ask funda-mental questions about the relevance and scope of the system of health care which they work for and perpetuate.

The PHC approach, though not complicated to understand, offers a new approach to the provision of health care. The newness of the approach can be shown by examining what a PHC approach to health education might be. Education is said to be an important part of any health service. Chapter Eight sets out to explore some of the far-reaching educational dimensions of PHC. If PHC is to have any chance of making inroads into the philosophy, policies and practice of health care, a new sort of health professional will be called for. This is the topic of the concluding chapter, Chapter Nine.

Western medicine is in an almost unassailable position of power and influence, its fundamental approach often seemingly beyond question. Yet PHC, David against Goliath, assails this position and asks basic questions. Whether they will be heard and used as constructive criticism is another matter.

Chapter One

The Why of Primary Health Care

Primary Health Care (PHC) is an approach to the planning of health services. In the last twenty years there has been a lively debate in Third World countries about the need for new approaches to health care, the validity of the PHC alternative, as well as about the scope of PHC activities and the consequences of the application of the PHC approach. PHC terminology appears in most national health policy documents. In Western countries, on the other hand, there is almost total ignorance about Primary Health Care on the part of health planners and health workers. This ignorance extends to both the meaning of the concept and examples of its practice. Many people have chosen to believe that Primary Health Care is to be equated with primary medical care. This is not the case and this book will argue that such ignorance cannot be allowed.

Western health services have well-established, not to say entrenched ways of understanding and practising health care. It has to be said, however, that even in these societies the policies and practice of health services are under question. The medical paradigm, our way of conceptualising health and health services, is changing, however slowly. It is commonplace to say that the world is shrinking, that what happens in one corner of the world can have an influence in another, distant part. In the world of health care, the Western mode of practising health care has exerted an enormous influence on health services in the rest of the world; this continues to be the situation. But the Third World is not only the receiver of ideas, it generates them as well. PHC is an example of this: the questions put to medical practice by the PHC approach in Third World countries and the issues it raises are relevant questions and important issues also for Western health services. Attempts to implement the PHC approach in the countries of Asia, Latin America and Africa have given rise to an important questioning of existing health services; the debate could be most useful in Western societies as well.

The words 'Primary Health Care' (PHC) are sometimes taken to mean health care at the periphery, or some programmes of extension or adjustment at the margins of the health services where these come into contact with communities. Primary *Health* Care then becomes equated with primary *medical* care or simple curative services with the addition, perhaps, of a prevention programme represented by an immunisation service or a water and sanitation programme. If it is only this, or becomes reduced to this, PHC is not particularly problematic or challenging. However, as presented by the international Conference of Alma Ata in 1978 and developed in a variety of contexts since, PHC is much more than an addition to existing health services, much more than primary medical care. It is a reorientation of all health services towards the health needs of communities, both local and national. This reorientation can have dramatic consequences on health care resources allocation, on priorities in planning and on the attitudes of health personnel. The vision of PHC presented by Alma Ata challenges many existing ways of thinking and practice in health services throughout the world.

The PHC approach rose out of the perceived inadequacies of conventional health care to meet the needs of people in Third World countries. It is an attempt to chart the way towards a more appropriate health care system. However, no one should claim that the PHC approach presents us with a magic formula to solve the numerous problems with the health services and of ill-health in these countries; what it does do is to point the way out of existing difficulties without pretending to have all the answers. What we do have, under the banner of PHC, is an opportunity to confront – and to begin to remedy – the imbalance of the past and to lay the foundations of a better health-care system for the future. What is more, it can now be said that the emergence on to the international scene of the arguments provided by PHC for a more appropriate needs-oriented health care system in developing countries can contribute to the movement towards a more appropriate health care system worldwide. The debate concerning PHC as promoted at Alma Ata in 1978 and the efforts to put its principles into practice since that time have put an alternative approach on the international health service agenda. The ideas and principles of PHC will not easily disappear; the issues that it raises demand to be addressed in all societies. The broad outlines of the PHC approach will be presented in Chapter Three. Before that, in order to grasp the full impact of the approach to health care set out by Alma Ata, it is necessary to have some idea of the soil out of which PHC ideas have grown.

In this chapter the question addressed will be: why has Primary Health Care come about? If PHC can be seen as an answer, what are the questions? What were the problems to which the PHC approach has been presented as a 'solution'? What was so wrong with the way things were in the health services in many countries that many people were led to put the case for and begin to implement, in however piecemeal a fashion, a radically alternative approach?

Health care systems based on the Western model have been so dominant, so widespread and so powerful, that they have often been treated as being above questioning. The medical culture which has arisen in the twentieth century has brought about a situation of acceptance of the status quo in medical matters. This is manifested, for example, in the way in which patients do not easily question the decisions of doctors, even in matters to do with their own health. Nurses, perhaps, might be questioned, if the patient feels confident or the nurse is approachable; but in general, medicine is enshrouded in a powerful mystique of science and status which inhibits accountability to patients or indeed anyone else in any direct manner. And although 'public' health doctors have a brief to work in/for/with communities, it is rare to find a situation where the same public is able to question the policies and practice of public health personnel.

Not only are individual health personnel by and large beyond questioning, the modern health care system is an institution which is almost as beyond critical examination as the Church was in the Middle Ages. It is even very difficult for politicians or political parties seeking to hold on to or acquire power to engage in any critique of the medical services. This is as true in Europe as it is in Asia, Africa or Latin America. In industrialised and non-industrialised countries alike, political parties of all persuasions can be seen treating the medical profession with extreme caution, not on account of an anxiety to hinder the great work of healing which the profession is engaged in, but out of fear of its strong political lobby. In 1990, General Ershad of Bangladesh, the then head of state, proposed a new national health policy which was based on the premise that all was not well with existing health provision and seemed to hold out hope of an improved health service offering a better deal for the majority of the population:

'The basic main thrusts of the policy are democracy and participation of the people ... raising public sector outlay in health and social welfare sectors to 10 per cent in phases, a commendable measure indeed in a region where public health sector allocation is often less than 1 per cent (*Link*, 1990: 2).

The medical profession objected to these new policy proposals and indeed seemed to have played a role in the downfall of the government proposing such changes. A major factor in the objections of the professionals appeared to have been the proposed restrictions on private practice (*idem*). In many countries there is still a powerful belief in the altruism of the medical profession which often removes it from the sphere of critical accountability.

It can be very difficult for many people to imagine that there are ways of thinking and doing health work other than those with which we have become familiar. It is also difficult for some to imagine that the present system is seriously flawed. There is a popular image of medicine as not only a notable and high-minded profession but one which is tackling the problems of ill-health in as scientific and concerned a manner as possible. Applied to the Third World, these beliefs contribute to the image of medicine in developing countries as consisting of the efforts of a few dedicated medical specialists to overcome the enormous tides of 'tropical' diseases and the ravages of ill-health which attack the defenceless (large) populations of these countries. Some health charities do not always do much to dispel this image when they propagate images of medical 'rescue' teams flying in to the aid of particular Third World countries beset with disease or disaster. Of course, rescue is sometimes necessary but both in such extreme cases and in the more habitual situations of ill-health the assumption is that the 'answer' to problems of ill-health lies in the medico-technical solution provided by expensively trained health personnel. In many situations this is simply not the case. The UNDP says that in the last decade of the twentieth century, 'More than a quarter of the world's people do not get enough food, and nearly one billion go hungry. 1.3 billion people still lack access to safe water. 2.3 billion lack access to sanitation' (UNDP, 1992: 14).

It is difficult to deny that the main answers to the problems of ill-health of millions of people lie outside the health sector and in other areas such as agriculture, education and sanitation. Many of the problems of ill-health facing Third World countries are not susceptible to medical interventions in the first place and what health care is called for can and should be delivered to those who need it by appropriately trained personnel as near and responsive to the community and its health needs as possible.

There is still much misplaced hope that medical systems can solve the world's health problems. The inherent problems of the way we conceptualise and therefore organise health services, what we can call the *medical model*, will be considered in the next chapter. It is enough to record here that it is the failure of this model of health care to meet the needs of the majority of people in so many countries which has given rise to the PHC movement.

The failure of the conventional system of health care

It is especially in so-called developing countries that the failures of the Western model of health care have become increasingly apparent over the last thirty or forty years. The process of 'modernisation' and development in these countries, including development of health services, has involved a long and destructive cultural invasion (Freire, 1970). When one group of people, or indeed a whole culture, experiences a systematic undervaluing of its beliefs, practices and view of the world and begins to see itself through the eyes of another oppressive culture, it can be said to have been culturally invaded. The process of colonisation of the Third World, to justify its very existence, was involved in such a systematic devaluing of all that was 'native'; in the area of beliefs Christianity was used to label much of what was local as 'superstitious', somehow irrational and inferior. In many areas of social organisation this contributed to the uncritical acceptance that 'West is best', with the undermining of the colonised people's sense of self-respect and dignity and a loss of a sense of pride in their own value system. In health service development what happened was often the total outward rejection of all traditional therapies and the proliferation of provisions based on a Western medical technical culture with no real attempt to match these to the major health needs of these countries. The colonisers knew what was 'good' for the colonised and this included what was good for their health. A considerable part of the message of what was good in health care came from denying the colonised to access of white services. A pattern of expectation was thus created, with distortions which remain to this day. The most obvious manifestation of the mismatch which can result from this medical colonialism is the skewed health budgeting which it inevitably brought. In countries where many of the diseases of the general population in terms of morbidity and mortality are those which are either preventable or easily treatable at the community level – and this is the case for most Third World countries – a large proportion of what little money there is for health often goes to buy Western medical technology for tertiary or secondary care.

That the basic health problems of many countries have not been addressed by considerable investment in institutions of tertiary care, and the concomitant neglect of community-level initiatives of cure and prevention, have been two of the major factors which have contributed to the emergence of the alternative approach to health care which we call Primary Health Care (PHC). Quite simply, despite considerable efforts to implement the Western health care system in Africa, Asia and Latin America, indicators of health status in these countries have continued to paint a very poor picture: UNICEF's annual statistics of global indices such as infant and maternal mortality continue to show high levels in many countries (UNICEF, 1991). It cannot be suggested that the form of health services adopted by Third World countries has been the major cause of ill-health in countries of the Third World, but the mismatch between service and need has been in evidence for several decades and contributes to the problem. In the 1960s and 1970s there was a growing frustration among many health workers with the seeming inability of conventional health care systems to impact significantly on the health status of large populations in these countries. PHC emerged as a strategy when these failures were becoming increasingly obvious. Frustrations with existing approaches led to criticism and, in some contexts, to changes. Innovative practices were tried with apparent success. The dimensions of some of these innovative practices were quite small (Newell, 1975) but the public health improvements in China which inspired some of the early PHC thinking were on a massive scale and involved, for example, the eradication of health-threatening pests, not in the first instance by *medicine*, but through social organisation and the use of local-level health workers, the famous barefoot doctors (Horn, 1971, Sidel and Sidel, 1982). For example, the mortality rate of infectious diseases in China declined from 116.30 per 100,000 in 1973–4 to 45.13 per 100,000 in 1982 (Huang, 1988:886). There is perhaps less enthusiasm now, even within the country itself, for the approach taken by China to promote health and eradicate disease and we can see there a definite move towards closer alignment with certain aspects of Western medicine. Ironically, the collective local commune organisations which were in some ways central to the grassroots organisation of primary health care in China were dismantled in 1978, the very year of the Conference of Alma Ata at which the Chinese approach to PHC was applauded (Huang, 1988). Recent commentators suggest, however, that the Chinese example of health care still offers a powerful alternative to the Western model.

Seen in this light, the PHC approach is an important part of the search for more appropriate health care for millions of people. The Indian Journal, *Health For The Millions* (VIHAI) which promotes PHC in that continent proclaims in its title, by implication, one of the major failings of the pre-PHC approach: health care in the old system was NOT for the millions but for the few. But the PHC approach starts from the position that not only are conventional forms of health care *insufficient* to meet people's health needs, they are also often *inappropriate*. Many Third World countries have tried with ever-diminishing success to expand the type of health care system they inherited at the time of independence to meet the needs of their populations. The problem is that their blueprint, the inherited model, was fundamentally flawed.

The inherited model: fatal inappropriateness

After the second world war many countries in Africa and Asia sought to rid themselves of colonial subjugation. With political independence, many countries found themselves committed to policies of social improvement. Both in education and in health (and indeed in other crucial areas like agriculture) considerable efforts were then made to expand services which had previously been largely restricted to the white minority and 'essential' workers in the colonial system. Inevitably, the new decision-makers and planners, aided by advisers from the West, expanded their social service systems along the lines of the model they had inherited. In Southern and Central American countries a similar process of modernisation was taking place with the dominant influence and role model being, this time, the United States and its value system.

Unfortunately, this model was exported to so-called developing countries at a time of colonial exploitation of which it was also an instrument (Doyal, 1979). Inevitably, the health systems reflected the values and beliefs of the colonisers. There were, of course, beneficial medical technologies in this inheritance. One can think, for example, of the knowledge of sterile operating techniques and, latterly, of antibiotics, to name only two major contributions. But there was much that was negative and destructive. We have already called attention to the attitude of misplaced, arrogant superiority towards most of what was local, however valuable. Indigenous healing systems were considered to be of no worth. In the spirit of cultural invasion, whereby the colonial power has a vested interest in belittling the values of the culture being colonised, traditional health care practices and beliefs were condemned and ridiculed. The tragedy of this is that a more detached view of these therapies now finds much that is of value in the holistic attitudes of traditional healers, much that complements the technical values of Western medicine, for example, the wisdom of Chinese understanding about health, including energy flows in the body and the related practice of acupuncture; modern Western attempts to 'de-medicalise' birth and provide more mother-centred birthing practices resembles very closely the caring provided by traditional birth attendants to African mothers. Many Western people, dissatisfied with the reductionist approach of their own 'traditional' therapies are turning to the health systems of the cultures their forefathers despised, in order to find a more holistic approach to healing and wholeness. But at the height of colonial territorial and cultural expansion, what happened was that indigenous people, recruited to Western-style health services, were obliged implicitly and sometimes explicitly to denounce their own heritage. The rejection called for by the colonial health authorities was total even in areas where the limitations of Western allopathic medical practice were obvious and indigenous therapeutic interventions had a record of success, as, for example, in many cases of mental illness. This unfortunate heritage remains even now when there is some effort to redress the balance and preserve what is of value in indigenous health systems (Bannerman et al, 1983).

The inappropriateness of the medical model inherited from the West by many countries is nowhere more apparent than in the work of most of the hospitals in these countries. A high proportion of the mortality and morbidity cases in institutions of health are related to easily preventable conditions or diseases, as is shown in the following table:

Some causes of mortality and morbidity at health centres in Zambia

Diagnosis	Mortality (% of total deaths)	In-patient (% of total admissions)
Measles	19.9	6.9
Malnutrition & Anaemias	15.5	4.4
Pneumonia	14.1	5.4
Malaria	11.3	19.5
Diarrhoea	9.9	7.7
Upper respiratory tract infections	2.4	6.3
Other abdominal cases	2.1	4.8
Injuries	1.1	5.4
Other pulmonary cases	0.8	1.8
Jaundice	0.8	0.3
Total	**77.9**	**62.5**

(Source: Government of Zambia, 1981:2–3)

These figures leave much untold, but they do indicate that in such institutions of curative care, and in a manner which is mirrored in health centres and hospitals throughout the Third World, many people are admitted and many die of conditions, which as the Government of Zambia itself had the courage to admit, could have been prevented or inexpensively treated nearer, or even in, the homes of the sufferers (Government of Zambia, 1981:3; Paine and Siem Tjam, 1988). Many of the diseases are diseases of poverty: measles is only a killer epidemic in the context of material and social deprivation. Malnutrition and infectious diseases work together, synergistically, especially in children. Although the figures are from the early 1980s, there is no indication that the health status of most Third World countries has drastically improved. Indeed, since that time another epidemic, AIDS, has come to add itself to the list and contributes to the decimation of populations, this time not the children, but the adult population.

In country after country of Africa, Asia and Latin America, the evidence points to the spending of considerable amounts of money on a health system which is not meeting the country's health needs because the focus is on treatment and cure within institutions. Instead of a health care system with a balance of 'promotive, preventive, curative and rehabilitative services' (Alma Ata, VII,2.), what is in evidence is a system with a distorted emphasis on curative care, the treatment of disease. In the words of the government of one country: 'Thus an expensive urban based medical system which relies on treatment rather than on prevention is clearly NOT an effective way to tackle the nation's health problems' (Government of Zambia, 1981:3).

When Ivan Illich (1975) denounced 'national health systems' as a misnomer, suggesting 'national disease systems' would be more accurate, he was referring to the current preoccupation of Western medicine with dealing with the manifestations of disease rather than the prevention of such conditions and the promotion of good health. This leads to an enormous emphasis on curative care and expenditure on institutions of treatment, like University Teaching Hospitals in capital cities. Illich's remarks have particular poignancy in poorer countries which spend such a high proportion of their limited resources on expensive treatment of preventable diseases in such institutions of tertiary care. Doctors and other health workers in hospitals which have high mortality figures from conditions which could have been prevented or treated at the village level, like diarrhoea and measles, are often acutely aware of the limitations of the treatment bias in Western-type health services. In many cases it was the experience of such inappropriateness which led to the first steps towards a Primary Health Care approach.

A recent report from health workers in South America shows that conditions by the late 1980s had not changed for the better:

> Recent data shows that 53.5% of the population (in this case, Peru) dies of infectious and endogenous diseases. Mortality rates due to contagious diseases have doubled in the last decade. Many of these (typhus, hepatitis and others) can be prevented by basic environmental sanitary actions, vaccination and improving the overcrowded conditions in which people are forced to live (Marshall and Yanz, 1988:5).

Unfortunately, health care has come to be confused with medical care. Many people are intellectually aware that hospitals in poor societies are treating the symptoms of poverty and an impoverished environment. Medical technology is not the answer to the diseases of poverty, cannot significantly alter the patterns of morbidity and mortality in many countries, yet it tends to consume whatever money there is for health. Like giving someone an expensive electric toothbrush to paint a house with, we are talking about the wrong tools for the job in hand. Institutions of tertiary care and the technology and personnel required to maintain them to 'international' standards use up an obscenely disproportionate share of the limited health budgets in all countries of the world. As Kennedy said of the British Health Service budget, 'the fact that an ever-increasing proportion (of this budget), now seventy percent, goes to hospitals could be said to be evidence of the failures of health care and how we perceive it' (Kennedy, 1981:32).

Kennedy is echoing the message of Illich, that the focus of our health system is on treatment of disease rather than on the promotion of health and prevention of illness. This is the voice of reason, not of fanaticism, and the case becomes even more pressing when we turn to poorer countries, often under pressure from their own medical profession and from influential groups within the country to keep to international standards but in a context of ever-diminishing resources and the spread of diseases of poverty.

If we take the example of Tanzania: it is a country which has been serious in its efforts to bring health care within reach of all its citizens. But even there the inherited emphasis on curative care, reported by a commentator on the country's health care system in the 1970s and unchanged since, shows the distortions caused by the priority given to tertiary care: ' ... the main government hospital ... consumed 14 per cent of the nation's total drug budget, compared with 15 per cent used by all the country's 220 health centres and 2,300 dispensaries' (Klouda, 1983: 59).

This pattern of distorted emphasis is repeated throughout the world, giving credence to David Morley's damning indictment of hospitals as 'disease palaces'. Felicity Savage King's assessment is just as perceptive: 'skills prisons' is how she describes many hospitals in Third World countries (Savage King, 1991), since within their walls are often contained much of the professional health work skills and the creative energies of the medical profession of many countries; these are kept away from the communities in real need of them and away from the tasks of prevention and education. Health care resources are separated from the health needs of the population by the model of health which underlines health planning. As we will see in the following chapter, the problem of the inappropriateness of health care in many Third World countries would not be resolved by more money in institutions of medicine: the model itself is seriously flawed and incapable of dealing with the task in hand.

Since hospitals are by and large located in urban areas, the majority of many populations do not have access to them and this often means no access to health care at all. 'Exceedingly poor access to health care, due in part to insufficient numbers of health facilities, particularly health posts (the most accessible source of health care for the bulk of the country's population). Inadequate supplies of essential drugs and long delays in drug procurement' (Carlaw, 1988:38): this is a description by USAID of the health service situation in Senegal but the author might well have been talking of the health services in many parts of Africa, Asia, or Latin America even today.

Inappropriate health care: the example of the management of malnutrition

The last few decades have witnessed dissatisfaction with existing health services and many attempts to widen the perspective and scope of conventional health care. There is clearly a very strong case for such an expanded perspective. If one takes the example of malnutrition and the attempts of the health systems of many Third World countries to manage this condition, the inappropriateness of these systems becomes strikingly apparent. At the core of the mismatch between need and service in this, as in many other cases, is the fact that the services are based on a narrow medical rather than a health view of ill-health. Malnutrition is widespread and of tragic proportions in many poorer countries. In the last twenty years the caloric intake per capita in some countries like Bangladesh and Chad has gone down (World Bank, 1990). Malnutrition is on the increase. More accurately, in most cases one should be speaking of 'undernutrition' in these countries, and, it could be argued, one should also consider speaking more directly of 'hunger' and 'starvation', since the basic problem is often lack of food and/or access to the possibility of acquiring it either through work on the land or other employment. Conventional health care tends to medicalise malnutrition, casting the problems of hunger and starvation in terms of their clinical symptoms and manifestations: 'stunting', 'marasmus', 'kwashiorkor' or 'protein energy malnutrition'. Of course, it is sometimes important to see the problem in this way, but it is just as important to remember that this clinical labelling provides us with only a partial view: the medical words can actually serve to hide or mask the ill-health conditions of poverty, in this case of hunger, by narrowing the focus of our attention. Many health workers involved in 'treating' malnutrition would readily acknowledge that the socio-economic and cultural aspects of hunger are as important as its clinical manifestations, yet 'health care' resources are almost inevitably turned towards interventions aimed at 'cure' and treatment. The medicalisation of malnutrition also serves the interest of those who do not wish for public examination of the social causes of hunger such as land distribution and unjust wage levels. In this way, even committed doctors and other health professionals can obscure the real issues of ill-health by focusing people's attention on the clinical symptoms of ill-health and their 'treatment', thereby deflecting attention away from structural causes of malnutrition such as those which we have mentioned.

Malnutrition and undernutrition are linked to many diseases of the Third World. The well-known (and, sadly, not frequently emulated) study of Serano and Puffer in 13 South American countries shows nutritional deficiencies as being an associated cause of all death in 47 per cent of children under three years of age and in around 60 per cent of deaths from diarrhoea, measles and infective and parasitic diseases in the same age group (Sanders, 1985:22). This confirms the conviction of many people working in the health field in numerous countries: behind the clinical conditions of many of their patients is an enormous reservoir of hunger and poverty. Measles and other infectious diseases only become killer diseases when associated with malnutrition and undernutrition, with hunger and starvation: 'Measles in Senegal is lethal because of the nutritional state of its victims. Sporadic village epidemics are known to kill upwards of 35 per cent of all village children under the age of five' (McEvers, 1980: 56).

The situation is replicated with distressing similarity in many poor countries, or at least in segments of their population. Most of the diseases presenting to medical institutions in these countries are diseases of poverty, often manifesting themselves in the first instance in undernutrition and susceptibility to infectious diseases, especially in the most vulnerable sector of any community, its children. This needs to be recognised by those responsible for the provision of health care and reflected in the interventions which are pursued. Children and the health-threatening conditions of poverty in which they live are therefore the legitimate focus of many health programmes. Children *are* the focus of many programmes, but unfortunately the context of poverty is often not. Of course, no health care system on its own can tackle the social economic conditions which are the root causes of these conditions. However, unless the health workers involved with the diseases of poverty widen their conventional perspective and take on board the wider causality of ill-health and the context of health and illness, they risk not seeing the real health problems of their patients; this can lead them to become involved in 'solutions' which actually do little to improve and even sometimes worsen the coping ability of those they are trying to help. Many people have witnessed health education programmes directed at women's ignorance of the benefits of protein or green vegetables, or brown bread for their children's growth. The medicalised perspective of malnutrition, with its focus on individual pathology or malfunctioning, finds a certain harmony with such a 'lifestyles' health education approach which acts as though the core of the problem lies in the ignorance of the mothers who are not giving their children the correct food to make them function properly. If the social causes of ill-health were seen as being just as important as the bio-physical ones, many causes of undernutrition and related infections would be acknowledged; this would involve the corollary that the mother's ability to influence and change the situation is severely limited. Whatever solution were suggested, there would be less danger of health professionals 'blaming the victim' (for further discussion of this point, see Chapter Eight).

Unfortunately, the victim-blaming approach goes along with and is reinforced by the dominant view of development in general. The 'modernisation' view of development, which is still the one which underlies most national programmes and international development aid, sees development as something which 'trickles down' from the 'developed' world or sector, through development workers to populations. Resistance to development as defined by experts is considered as backwardness: professionals must learn to recognise obstacles to the diffusion of progress and to be prepared to tackle these obstacles (Rogers, EM, 1969). According to this way of seeing things, the problems lie within – within the individuals, within their 'apathy' or 'perceived limited good' or their 'fatalism' or their culture. Development workers, in such a perspective of the problem, must learn how to tackle these internal deficiencies of their 'clients'. It is not hard to see the convenient alliance between such a view of the need for development and a system of health care based on curative care. In the world of development, this view of 'internal deficiencies' has been strongly criticised, especially in Latin America (Macdonald, 1986). As Rodney says in the context of Africa, much of what is conventionally described as the causes of underdevelopment, are often actually the consequences of underdevelopment and make sense only when seen in the context of the impact of the exploitation of Africa, Asia and Latin America by the West (Rodney, 1972); the squalor of the cities of the Third World (Harpham, 1989) and the poor nutritional status of plantation workers in Africa and Asia (Laing, 1986) are two examples of situations which have been seen as causing underdevelopment but are clearly, in another perspective, caused by it. For both development and health professionals it is often convenient to ignore questions which oblige consideration of the wider issues of history and social and economic causes, especially exploitation. As a result, the focus continues to be on the within perspective, on internal deficiencies.

A wider perspective leads the health worker into the social and economic realm and she or he might feel safer not to go down this road. The proven links between poverty and malnutrition and between malnutrition and infectious diseases, however, call for a wider perspective on problem and solution. The facts are that malnutrition precipitates common infections and these, in their turn, can precipitate malnutrition. As UNICEF says, in many situations, neither condition alone would usually cause death, but together they can be fatal, especially to children (UNICEF, 1984: 23). This situation of the 'synergistic' relationship of infections and malnutrition is a tragic and inescapable part of the experience of many health workers and has led them to question the adequacy of the medical framework in which they have been formed to deal with such a situation.

Malnutrition as a condition with its roots in people's poverty is certainly a widespread problem. What one report says about food and income in Guatemala has its parallels in many countries: 'Income determines consumption. Half of the total population of Guatemala consumes only 50 per cent of the calories necessary to maintain normal physical growth and to replace the energies consumed in work' (O'Sullivan 1980: 53).

Many people are living on the edge of starvation; by any criterion, this must be seen as a tragic situation of non-health and one which the medical systems of many Third World countries are inadequate to tackle. The causes of malnutrition often lie outside the control of individual families and even countries. People have sometimes tried to 'develop', following the road of modernisation we have already spoken about and actually found themselves in a worse-off economic situation with impaired nutritional status. A study by Jakobsen in the Southern Highlands of Tanzania even attributes an increase in malnutrition to the growth of the monetary economy, with nutritional levels highest in those families who had not 'modernised' but stayed outside the monetary economy in the subsistence farming sector (Klouda, 1983: 56).

As a result, health workers, faced with the problems arising from malnutrition, find themselves having to deal with conditions which arise out of the social and economic environment and, more specifically, from the poverty of their patients. The perspectives and tools with which the medical profession are supposed to deal with this situation are biomedical and individual-oriented. This is true in all countries, of course, but the mismatch is more obvious in poor countries which seem caught in a spiral of rising costs for medical technology which at best will satisfy the medical needs of a few. There is not much scientific glamour about water and sanitation programmes and anti-poverty campaigns. Institutional health care, which may have seemed like the solution at a time when its services were confined to the colonial minority and denied to the indigenous majority, has its attractions. It seemed like development to expand such health care institutions; hospitals seem like signs of progress. But the inappropriateness of such 'solutions' is ever more obvious. It was growing dissatisfaction with this gap between problem and solution, between the health needs of vast populations and the kind of medical services available which created the drive for alternatives, alternatives which would stress prevention of disease and the promotion of health and health-sustaining environments. By the 1970s the time was ripe for a new approach.

And so we have the emergence of the Primary Health Care perspective. The failure of the existing system was patently obvious. It should not, of course, be hoped that PHC can, with the wave of a wand produce a new model of health care which will replace the existing one and solve all the problems that have been spoken about. What is being said is that PHC emerged on to the international stage when many of the failings of the dominant paradigm of health care were being exposed. PHC is part of the search for a new model of health care which incorporates the advantages of modern medicine but which seeks to include a wider vision of health and health care into its system.

In Third World countries the limitations of the approach of health services were acutely felt by many health workers: there is the enormous task of dealing with the diseases of poverty, of malnutrition and the infections which are associated with it, especially for poor communities. There is need for a health care system which is both curative and preventive. There is need for the health professionals to acknowledge their limitations in dealing with these problems and to show a readiness to work with other sectors which promote health, like agriculture and education. There is a need for all professionals working in the public domain to work with communities, to work in partnership with them in the building of healthy environments. These needs are the basis of the call for a new approach.

But the obstacles are many. For example, there is an expectation that capital cities have gleaming high-rise hospitals offering 'international' standards of treatment. This expectation of medicine has entered into popular consciousness and in many societies people have come to confuse big hospitals with good health services. The model of health care which has come to dominate the world has in it a great emphasis on medical technology and medical science and this requires the costly production of medical technologists, medical scientists. What is the medical framework which lies behind the inappropriateness of health services? The next chapter will attempt to understand better this medical 'model' which exerts such a great influence on the health services of so many countries and whose limitations have brought about the demand for a new way of thinking and acting in health care.

Chapter Two

The Medical Model as Obstacle

The Western model of health: an engineering model

The Western medical model has been described as an engineering model (McKeown, 1976: 6; Engel, 1976: 131). The analogy of the body as a machine and the doctor as the medical scientist/engineer has proved useful to the development of certain aspects of medical care, especially in crisis interventions and in the treatment of acute clinical disorders. But the engineering analogy *is* only an analogy and the complexities of human health and ill-health in all societies, and not just in poorer countries, are such that health care and health services cannot be adequately contained within such a framework. The attempt to manage ill-health along lines dictated by this framework has produced some of the distortions in health care dealt with in the previous chapter, especially the tendency to focus most effort and resources on the treatment/curative dimensions of health care. One of the greatest drawbacks of the medical culture that has grown up with the engineering model is the removal of the patient or the community from any situation of control in the encounter with the medical profession. 'Disease' tends to be seen, by professional and lay-person alike, as something 'objective', somehow *in* the individual or in the community, but separable from them, waiting to be identified and dealt with by the medical profession.

Although written some years ago, Arthur Keith's book, *The Engines Of The Human Body*, is a fine illustration of the medical culture fostered by the engineering model of health. The body is a fascinating machine, he says, mysterious and complex:

> There is a machine which every one of us has to drive

> morning, noon and night, day by day, year in and year
> out, until the end of life's journey ... Some (man-made)
> machines are wonderfully made ... but not one of them,
> not even the most intricate, is so hard to understand as
> the human machine — your body and mine (Keith,
> 1919:1).

Keith goes on to share with his reader his enthusiasm for medical
research, focused on ever-increasing knowledge of the human
machine with the greater accuracy of vision provided by the
microscope:

> Up to the year 1839 medical men always wrote and spoke
> of man's body in this way (as if it were a single machine)
> ... After 1839 it was no longer possible for them to look on
> it in this simple manner. At this date the microscope
> became sufficiently powerful to reveal the secret struc-
> ture of the tissues which form the body. Skin, bone, hair,
> nails, nerves, muscles and brain were, one after the other,
> shown to be made up of minute living units or cells closely
> set together in hordes or masses (Keith, 1919: 326).

The body, then, is this wonderfully complex machine, or
combination of machines, becoming increasingly more understandable through microscopic inspection. Keith's assumption is
that this increased understanding will reveal the causality of
disease to the medical scientist and chart the way to a healthier
society. The world of medical science has developed enormously
since Keith's time, largely in the direction he hoped for and in
some areas has contributed greatly to human health. But this
progress has done little to remove many of the colossal mountains
of suffering and ill-health which exist in the societies of the Third
World with their patterns of communicable diseases often rooted
in poverty. The model and the systems it informs also increasingly
fails to deliver in Western societies where the common pattern of
disease in the community at large is often one of psychosocial
problems and diseases of an ageing population: '... there are
increasing numbers of the elderly who suffer from chronic diseases
of old age. Cardiovascular diseases, cancer, mental disorders,
rheumatisms, arthritis and permanent disability are the major
health problems among the elderly (Maglacas, 1984: 86).

It would be irrational to invest in medical science great
expectations for the removal of this suffering, either of the
diseases of poverty in the Third world, or of psychosocial and

degenerative diseases in Western societies. Nevertheless, the allure of the myth that there is a medical answer to the problems of the world's health continues to be a most powerful one; Keith's fascination with the microscopic view of the human body/machine is still at the forefront of medical science:

> It may take many thousands of years more, but I am certain that if we apply ourselves to its study as anatomists and physiologists have done and are doing, the time will come when we shall understand the human body – how it feels, sleeps, wakes, plays, and works – just as perfectly as we know the machinery of the steam engine which pulls a railway train or the internal-combustion engine which drives a motor bicycle (Keith, 1919: 3).

That is to say, the complexity of the human body – and its ills – will be understood and become treatable (and, presumably, a new era of health will emerge) by the applying to the problems of ill-health the sophisticated technology of medicine which science will make available. There is an increasingly global medical culture which has as one of its foundation stones the often unquestioned optimistic view that the development of more sophisticated medical technology will improve the status of human health. This is an assumption which has been proved false in many societies and for many conditions of human health and well-being. To reduce ill-health to an area susceptible of technical fixes is to ensure that health services will fail in the way they have done so dramatically in poorer countries and increasingly also in developed societies.

Medicine did not always have such a narrow view in Western society. The early 19th century had seen, in what has been called the era of public health, a growing understanding of the wider circles of causality of human health and ill-health: the influence of social, cultural and economic and environmental factors on human health was accepted and acted upon. The impact of water and sanitation on the spread or prevention of infectious diseases was understood. Great advances were made in this era. But gradually the work of 'public health' became separate from the work of physicians; 'scientific medicine' came to mean the kind which Keith represents and idealises. This separation continues in most countries of the world. Sadly, the 'engineering' model of health which dominates the world of medicine today is not an engineering one of the public health kind but one focused on the individual human body conceived of as a machine. Medical attention had been distracted away from other, wider issues just as important in the understanding of human health and illness as individual bio-pathology. The context in which individual human beings live out their lives has a significant impact, either negative or positive, on their health: their emotional state, the support of their family and friends, the physical environment, their income and a whole variety of other 'circles' all influence health, but the engineering model tends to overlook them in the name of 'science'. The focus is that of the microscope rather than what we might call the 'macroscope'.

In a chapter entitled 'In The Repairing Shops' Keith carries the engineering analogy further: 'We medical men', he says, 'are wayside repairers of the human machines which break down on the road of life'. Of course, it has to be said that much excellent caring – and repairing – has gone on under the inspiration of this vision of sick human beings as broken-down vehicles and doctors as the mechanics waiting to help and repair. What is in question is whether this view has outlived its useful life and needs to be supplemented, if not supplanted, by an understanding of health and disease which allows for a wider causality and would lead to a different approach to solutions.

Commentators like McKeown would suggest that the concep-tualisation of medical practice as a form of scientific biological engineering begins from the very start of most medical training: 'Physics, chemistry and biology are considered to be the sciences basic to medicine; medical education begins with the study of the structure and function of the body, continues with examination of disease processes and ends with clinical instruction on selected sick people' (McKeown, 1976: 6).

The world of the wider circles of causality of disease and especially of health, the world of the 'macroscope', are relegated to marginalised courses of 'social science'. The principal focus is indisputably on biological pathology:

> Western medicine has long viewed the body as a machine that could be analysed in terms of its parts ... With its focus upon pathology, the present medical model attri-butes the ultimate origin of illness to biological factors ... thus the patient is viewed much like an automobile, both being machines requiring repair (Pelletier, 1979: 31).

There is not much indication that the medical profession sees its limited vision as an obstacle in the way of appropriate health care.

The engineering model is alive and well. In the UK, motor cars of more than three years are by law subjected to an 'MOT' (Ministry of Transport) test to check for their road-worthiness or lack thereof. It is quite common for doctors and nurses examining young children in their first weeks of life to check all the limbs and reactions of the child, often without any collaboration with the passive parent, and to declare, 'OK, she's passed her MOT'. Such medical workers can become accustomed to seeing their task as being that of a mechanic, often without the slightest suspicion that they may, by this way of looking at both the reality of the child and their role as health worker, be limiting their vision of human health and disease to a perspective which misses much of what sustains or threatens the well-being of the patient. The engineering model has its uses but it can induce tunnel-vision and needs to be enlarged.

The engineering model of health care can be fairly described as being a reactive rather than a proactive one. The emphasis is on waiting for something to go wrong; the sufferer then approaches the medical professional, the problem is diagnosed and dealt with. In this sense, medical science, says Kennedy, 'is concerned with reaction, response to ills which already ail the sufferer ... what we have ... is a system of medicine which responds, which waits to pick up the broken pieces – a form of medicine, in short, concerned with illness, not health (Kennedy, 1981: 28).

Another and equally unflattering way of describing this mode of operation of conventional medicine, would be to describe it as the 'fire brigade' approach: illness in the community is like the outbreak of a fire and the role of the medical profession is to douse the fire. Many doctors would resent this description of their work, yet in many cases it is rather difficult to deny the preponderantly reactive mode of operation of modern medical practice. In industrialised countries there is more spent on hospitalised treatment of cardiovascular disease, for example, than on its prevention. In countries of the Third World the consequences are sometimes obscene; we saw in the last chapter that the disease pattern in many of these countries is of diseases of poverty often amenable to treatment and even prevention when dealt with early on at a level of care near the community. However, most of the scarce money available for health services goes on the reactive model we are describing, waiting with its costly personnel and equipment to 'pick up the broken pieces'.

In this way, an understanding of the perspectives of health care encouraged by the engineering model helps to illuminate the misfit already spoken about between the health needs of the so-called developing countries and their systems of health services, based on the Western medical model. A similar mismatch between need and provision in Western societies has also been pointed out. In the last chapter we gave the example of the common problem of malnutrition. With this, as with many other common conditions, instead of prevention and treatment at a local level with a community focus, most countries have a treatment/curative approach which is costly and often urban-based. As we have seen, the biological perspective of this focus on treating the symptoms of complaints tends to bring the attention of the health services on to the individual physiology of the patient and exclude consideration of the socio-economic context in which she or he operates. Prevention and education dimensions, likewise, when they are addressed, tend to focus on individual behaviour, with the health professional exhorting individuals to change that behaviour, to alter their lifestyles. In recent years there has been a major focus in Western health systems on education to promote healthier lifestyles. This is entirely consistent with the medical model and an emphasis on the individual's responsibility for maintenance of his/her body. In the early 1990s in the UK, government advice on the 'Health of the Nation' included advertisements in daily newspapers encouraging readers to send for their copy of the 'maintenance manual': instructions on how to better care for the machine which is the human body. Of course, there are things which many people can do to improve their health and save 'garage' costs, but there are many factors beyond individual responsibility. To imply otherwise, and the medical model lends itself to such a view, is to distort with partial truth.

The limitations of this narrow focus of health education has received some attention in the context of Western societies (Rodmell and Watt, 1986; Research Unit in Health and Behavioural Change, 1989). The health education focus on lifestyle seems particularly inappropriate in countries and communities where environment and poverty are clearly important contributory factors to disease. Its limitation will be further discussed in Chapter Eight. Research in British cities has demonstrated the links between poor housing and ill-health (Martin et al, 1987). Tenants' associations have struggled, sometimes armed with such research, to challenge this situation and have the housing improved, often against great odds. The medical world, instead of seeing this movement as a necessary one for the improvement of people's health and supporting it, can allow its medical engineering blinkers to disavow any role for health workers in this struggle for health. The symptoms can be treated by medicine, but when medical interventions are accompanied by exhortations to changes in behaviour, it is understandable that these fall on resistant ears. As one tenant organiser put it, 'Don't come and tell us about brown bread and jogging: the problem is the bad housing we are forced to live in. Our health will improve when the housing does' (McCormack, 1991). The limitations of the medical model are manifest in all societies. Its limited vision of the causes for ill-health narrows its perspective on solutions to these problems as well: 'Very many of the people to whom we are readily prepared to ascribe the status "ill" find themselves ill because they are poor, grow up in bad housing, eat poor food, work, if at all, at depressing jobs, and generally exist on the margin of survival' (Kennedy, 1981: 42).

Those formed in the engineering model of health might give notional assent to such a causality of disease but in practice it will not influence their diagnosis or prognosis, their work practice. 'Yes, but so what?' may well be their reply to such criticisms, these cannot be our concerns. And so are revealed the tragic limitations of a health care model which is in fact a medical model.

Kennedy was talking about Britain, but his remarks on the social context and causes of ill-health apply to most countries of the world. The links between poverty and ill-health are well-documented (Townsend and Davidson, 1982), although such links do not often alter the medical vision or generate alternative approaches. In the early 1990s an editorial in the British Medical Journal reminded us: 'Eliminate poverty and health improves, everyone acknowledges that as a truth for the inhabitants of Third World shanty towns. What recent research in social medicine has now shown is that health continues to improve progressively as people get wealthier' (British Medical Journal, 1990).

These clearly-established links between economic status and health tend to be obscured by the tunnel-vision induced by the engineering model of health care which is now dominant throughout the world. The training of health workers as medical scientists or medical engineers leads to a focus on biological pathology, with what has been seen to have broken down in the individual human body, to the practical exclusion of the wider causes of ill-health in society and the economic world.

The health worker cannot, of course, be expected to take responsibility for the alleviation of the poverty which breeds disease or the poor environment, neither for the lack of care in society for an ageing population. What is important is to realise the limits of medicine and to ascribe to it its proper place in the amelioration of the condition of human health. There must be an acknowledgement of the vital role of curative care, of treatment, but as part of a health-care approach, not the entire approach.

The body as a machine: passive patients and male doctors

Throughout the world the public is now conditioned to see health and ill-health as being the medical profession's business: we submit ourselves into their hands rather as we hand over a machine to be repaired by a mechanic. PHC, however, proclaims 'participation' as one of its key strategies: people becoming actively involved in the health care process not just through compliance with the instructions of the health profession but in some form of partnership or collaboration with them. The public is not accustomed to this role; neither is the health profession. The engineering model of health care has influenced the way the relationship between the public and the health professional is understood by both 'partners'. The engineering model encourages a passive, non-participatory role for the lay person and an active, decision-making role for the health professional. Most medically-trained workers who try to work in a participatory manner find themselves in difficulties. It should not be assumed that this is due to some fatal inevitable autocratic trait in the personality of the individuals concerned. It probably has much more to do with a mode of operation inculcated from the first days of training as medical scientists. Once health workers become more conscious of the engineering model which has formed them, they have the chance of adopting an approach which retains what is good in this formation while attempting to unlearn certain approaches which are not conducive to people's participation (Macdonald, 1982).

The engineering model of medical care is profoundly rooted in Western culture and is often traced back to the philosopher, Descartes. Descartes saw the body as an intricate machine regulated by the law of physics; a machine which can be taken apart and reassembled if we learn to understand its functioning properly (McKeown, 1976). The height of medical progress in this perspective would be organ transplants, seen by some as the apex of health-care achievement in our time. Such operations certainly represent considerable technical achievement: individuals with defective parts can have these replaced and the contribution of some of these interventions should not be slighted. The focus of intervention, however, is at a stage when the condition is already developed beyond the level of prevention. As we have said, the model is reactive rather than proactive. If we take the example of heart transplants and coronary by-passes, the dramatic nature of the interventions and the popular interest these often arouse can obscure the fact that expenditure in this direction inevitably diverts funds away from other areas like prevention which are also very important but do not call for dramatic surgery and are less 'media-genic'. One medical commentator and critic of what he sees as an undue emphasis on transplants says, 'I have no doubt that thousands of people who have died of heart disease in the last few years would still be alive today if the money spent on transplantation had been spent instead on preventive medicine. The simple fact is that most heart disease is preventable' (Coleman, 1988: 160). The option for the high-tech medical intervention involved in cardiac surgery is consistent with what we have described as the engineering model of health care.

For Descartes, the human body was a machine. A very complex one, certainly, and one created by God, but a machine nevertheless; he says that careful consideration will help us 'consider this body as a machine, which, having been made by the hands of God, is incomparably better ordered, and has in it more admirable movements than any of those invented by men' (Descartes, [1637], 1968: 73). The Cartesian understanding of the body as a machine which, though vastly more complicated than a watch, could nevertheless be opened out and understood in the same way, has helped the development of health sciences. But, as we have said, the vision has its own limitations. Cartesian scientific materialism is reductionist in that it tends to reduce what is complex – the human reality – to its perceivable parts. The consequences of this reductionism have perhaps never been better described than by Bannerman, speaking of the medical model which resulted from this perspective:

Its method [that of the science coming from Descartes' approach] was to break up complex phenomena into their component parts and deal with each one in isolation. In diagnosis this approach resulted in the search for a single cause; in pharmacology the search was for an active principle that could be isolated; and in the doctor–patient relationship the search for an efficient treatment of the physical causes of the symptoms tended to exclude any serious interest in the complexity of the life situation in which the patient was immersed (Bannerman et al, 1983: 11).

The medical focus, as it discovers more and more of the intricacies and complexities of the human machine, has inevitably to become a specialised vision, as no one discipline, let alone individual, could possibly keep up with the vast amount of information which is being generated (Mahler, 1975).

The engineering model also leads to dualism, the division of the human being into discrete entities of body and soul. For Descartes, the soul is distinct from the body which it informs: 'I imagined it was something extremely rare and subtle, like a wind, flame or vapour, which permeated and spread through my most substantial parts' (Descartes [1641] 1968: 104). The division of human reality in this way: body/soul, has persisted in one form or another in medical thinking until our day and, however poetically expressed, is a simplistic, dualist and inherently deficient understanding of human reality. It is shown to be deficient and runs into difficulties as an explanation of this reality when dealing, for example, with some aspects of what is known as 'mental' illness or conditions described as 'psychosomatic'. The complex, composite nature of human reality is being increasingly recognised and a dualist model is proving inadequate. Kennedy (1981) questions our allowing the 'labelling' of who is to be considered mentally ill to the medical profession trained in such a way of thinking. Newton points to what must be acknowledged at least as predisposing conditions of much mental illness in the social and psychological context of the sufferers: 'Rates of effective psychoses ... are frequently above average in widows, refugees, military conscripts, inadequately prepared immigrants, mothers whose children have left home and residents of districts where social interaction is weak, but low in religious communities and during secular movements such as the student protests of the late 1960s' (Newton, 1988: 25). The world of mental health is therefore obliged to go beyond the restrictions of the bio-engineering model and incorporate wider circles of causality of ill-health. It is sometimes from the discipline of psychiatry that demands for a more comprehensive model of health and health care have come.

In non-Western societies health traditions have a lively consciousness of the *oneness* of what the West has come to see as body–mind division and so of the spiritual dimension of health and disease. The imposition of Western understanding of 'mental health' on these cultures of health care is one of the most significant mismatches brought about by the colonial period. One of the least-tackled challenges of the health services in the Third World must lie in the dialogue called for between those formed in Western psychiatric approaches and indigenous understanding of mental well-being in order to find the 'socially acceptable methods and technology' (Alma Ata) needed in culturally appropriate health services (Bannerman et al, 1983).

One other characteristic of the Western medical model is the masculine domination of the health profession. Specialised engineering, and so medical engineering, is generally considered to be a male domain. Not only is medicine being revealed as a way of men exercising control over women (Ehrenreich and English, 1978), but when women do have a role in the medical process it is mostly an ancillary one. Often they are ascribed the nursing role; it is perhaps not too crude to say that in the engineering model of health care men do the 'health' (understood as medicine) and women do the 'care'. The medical profession can reinforce oppressive attitudes to women; on that topic, several Indian commentators have this to say:

> The medical profession also pays little attention to the health problems of working-class women, who form the majority of women in India. The health problems of these women are mainly related to their poverty and their inferior status within Indian society. However, health services attempt to reach these women only when they are pregnant, delivering or lactating' (Sathyamala et al, 1986: 108).

The inequalities experienced by women – and indeed by other groups – in terms of health services will be more fully addressed in Chapter Seven, but it is worth noting here that the same Indian commentators go on to point out that, in their own, as in many societies, the medical perspective is 'on either helping women to perform their reproductive function properly or in controlling their fertility' and in either case the medical profession reflects the dominant views in society. The fact that in most societies women are the custodians and promoters of health in families and communities is a basic fact sometimes of supreme importance in terms of the prevention of disease and enhancement of health of families. Yet, because these factors belong to circles of concern lying beyond the bio-physical, they tend to be overlooked by the engineering model of health and at best 'relegated' to the domain of social work.

Medical vision or health vision? Microscope or macroscope?

If we consider humans as being involved in, and even part of, a series of interacting systems which impact on health, we can identify systems of which the units get ever smaller: a system of organs, then of cells, then of the atomic particles which constitute these cells, etc. This can be seen as a series of concentric circles. We can also conceive of human beings as parts of wider systems: circles which consist of other people, families, socio-economic groups, cultures, etc. An understanding of the influence of both the inward circles and the outward circles is imperative in order to assess the health of the human person, no matter how health is defined. A mother presents a child who is suffering from diarrhoea and malnutrition. If we are interested in treating and preventing the condition in a long-term perspective, the anxieties of the mother about her child's health, as well as her family situation and economic condition and her culturally-induced beliefs are often just as important for helpful diagnosis and prognosis as knowing whether the child had four or five loose stools on a particular day and whether we should describe the malnutrition as *kwashiorkor* or *marasmus* or a combination of them both, or indeed, by some other label. As we saw in the previous chapter, the outward-reaching circles of which the child is a part are clearly of supreme importance in terms of healing and sustaining health. Yet the doctor, in almost any country of the world, is trained to believe that in the few minutes he has with the patient his task is to diagnose the 'problem' and prescribe for it. The engineering model of health turns the vision of the doctor towards the inward-reaching circles, towards the intra-organic and intra-cellular in order to discover what is causing the malfunction. In such a view of ill-health, 'medical work' tends to be seen in terms of the search for an appropriate medical intervention at the micro-biological level. This has influenced even the prevention side of modern medicine, so that vaccination – a clear medical intervention – becomes the major strand of preventive work, to the obvious neglect of environmental, educational and even nutritional activities.

Zola's analogy of the river, as popularised by McKinley (1979) offers an apt description of the distortions possible in health services as a consequence of the 'microscopic' view of health and illness leading to the focus on technico-medical solutions. The river is the tide of sickness into which the physician plunges to rescue people without having the time to understand and do anything about the factors which are pushing the people into the river in the first place, for example, their socio-economic conditions. McKinley's effort to help health workers 'refocus upstream' is part of the movement from microscope to macroscope born out of the frustration with the reactive engineering model of health care.

The setting was the first training of village health workers organised by the present writer. A role play was asked of the participants, to show the differing approaches of traditional and modern medicine. The situation to be role-played was that of a mother whose first child had died, seeking help for her sick new child, first from the traditional healer and then from a modern doctor. To the traditional healer the woman explained her difficult situation; they sat on the floor together and he consoled her with comments on the pressures she must feel from relatives and her high level of anxiety. He consulted the spirits and offered herbal remedies and a warning against a certain member of her extended family. The same participants then played out the encounter of the same mother with the modern health services. This was done with no hint of criticism, indeed the players, village health workers in training, were playing out the kind of role they aspired to. 'Bring me a white coat and a stethoscope,' said the 'doctor'. He sat on a chair behind a table. 'Next, please,' he said, and unwrapped the bundle the woman placed on his table; he used his stethoscope and thermometer and reached for anti-malarial drugs: 'Give so many of these to the child and come back if she doesn't improve,' only then looking at the mother. 'Next, please,' he said. The engineering model of health care is alive and well.

That the focus of health work is on what we have called the 'inner circles', those accessible to the world of the microscope, in the human experience of health and ill-health rather than the 'outer circles', those requiring a 'macroscope' can be shown not only by anecdotal evidence but from the nature and focus of most health, or rather, medical research. Scientific medical research and journals to disseminate it abound: 'There are so many medical journals in existence that a new scientific paper is published somewhere in the world every twenty eight seconds. There are 6,000 medical journals regularly being published around the world' (Coleman, 1988: 110).

It might be reasonable to hope that this enormous output of

medical energy would bring about a parallel diminishment in the tide of human suffering and an improvement in the quality of life for many of the world's inhabitants or at least would concern itself in a large measure with such a task. But this does not seem to be the case. The focus of the research in these journals is certainly on the 'inner circles', investigations of the application of some technical intervention in the domain of biology or bio-chemistry. Some commentators say of this situation that even in considerations of life circumstances and their impact on physical illness,

> The underlying model in most of this body of research is socio-biological ... That is, it assumes that social and psychological events which people experience, are experienced by the body as a machine, in terms of endocrinal and neuromechanisms ... It is basically a mechanical model of disease ... which is extended beyond mere internal physiological models to include the outside social environment of individuals (Research Unit in Health and Behavioural Change, 1989: 13).

Again, the consequences of such a focus are saddest in the countries of the Third World. The medical profession of these countries, if they wish to gain status and acclaim, rarely do so by tackling the well of suffering in their countries; those involved in this endeavour often go largely unnoticed or are labelled as extremists, especially if they look at historical and economic causes of present disease patterns. Prestige in medicine goes to those who have followed a narrow specialisation of disease and have published in the journals of medicine. The reservoir of poverty and disease is seen to be the domain of charity and the Mother Theresas of this world, not the burning, over-riding concern of medical science or of medical services.

Linked to the vision of the engineering model of therapy is what has been called the 'doctrine of specific aetiology'. In his historical overview of the development of Western medicine, René Dubos has traced the movement away from disease understood as lack of harmony (the understanding of 'pre-scientific' times), to the present position through the pioneering work of Louis Pasteur and Robert Koch. Our present policies and perspectives have been enormously influenced by the demonstrations of these scientists that some diseases could be produced by introducing a single specific factor, a virulent micro-organism, into a healthy animal. Dubos acknowledges the achievements which followed in the wake of these advances and which he sees as constituting the bulk of modern medicine. But he goes on to point out the limitations of this 'doctrine of specific aetiology': 'Few are the cases in which it has provided a complete account of the causation of diseases ... search for *the* cause may be a hopeless pursuit because most disease states are the indirect outcome of constellation of circumstances rather than the direct result of single determinant factors' (Dubos, 1959).

Although in theory the notion of disease as an outcome of a constellation of circumstances might be acknowledged, a multi-rooted aetiology, Western allopathic medicine, in the form with which it meets the public, still continues along the road of specific aetiology, despite the limitations of this path. One of the reasons why this rather simplistic view still has such influence on the day-to-day practice of medicine must surely be the congruence of this doctrine with the convenient idea that every specific disease has a specific remedy: a pill for every ill. Pharmaceutical products have come to be seen, often by public and practitioner alike, as the tools of choice of the medical profession.

The engineering model and its tools: pharmaceuticals

Much of the budget of the health services in many countries goes on salaries of doctors. Much also goes on the provision of drugs to institutions of care. A considerable proportion of family budgets in poor countries goes on buying the drugs which doctors have prescribed for their health. The scientific-engineering model of health accords a very special role to pharmaceutical products, seen as the essential tools of doctors as engineers. WHO has shown the importance and feasibility of a rational essential drugs policy. This policy accords a real place to pharmaceutical products in what can be described as a holistic approach to health care: drugs are a necessary part of a health-care system, which should encompass curative, rehabilitative, prevention and education programmes. The provision of essential drugs has always been considered as an essential 'component' of PHC programmes (Declaration of Alma Ata, VII, 3). But in the perspective of PHC and of WHO's Essential Drugs Strategy, the use of these drugs should be regulated by the health needs of the community rather than by the perspectives of pharmaceutical producers, especially their need to maximise profits. The Essential Drugs Programme, which offers countries guidelines and support in pursuing a balanced drugs-purchasing policy, has, of course, run into difficulties from those who profit from the proliferation of pharmaceutical products on the 'free' market. In 1982, one month after the government of Bangladesh had banned the use of 1,700 unwanted drugs, Western governments, including the USA, under pressure from the multinational drug companies, obliged the Bangladeshi government to set up a committee to review the new law (Medawar, 1984: 19). Such pressure can be very strong in situations where Third World countries often find themselves unable to take up a position of genuine dialogue or equality when faced with Western countries since many are caught in the web of debt-servicing and aid-dependency. The work of individuals like Charles Medawar and organisations like Social Audit have been brave Davids in face of the giant Goliaths of international and even national pharmaceutical companies in calling attention to the links between governments and such companies and between the latter and the medical profession: '... governments usually have a strong vested interest in the commercial performance of the home drug industry. Governments gain from companies' success – from taxes and export earnings ... Governments in general also rely strongly on political support from doctors and from drug companies and therefore tend to appease them' (*ibid*: 19).

The combination of the drug companies' need to sell and the doctors' need to prescribe is a powerful one. Pharmaceutical products, drugs, fit well into the model of 'scientific' health interventions: 'The model assumes that virtually all illnesses are due to measurable biochemical mishaps ... a chemical can then be tailored to reverse, ameliorate or prevent the biochemical failures ... The dream of 'one pill for one ill' has always been behind the medical-scientific model' (Fabricant and Hirschorn, 1987: 207).

'A pill for every ill' is not just a slick slogan, it represents a very real and – if one may say – unhealthy state of affairs. Of course, the public in many countries has now been conditioned to expect such a technical fix for their ill-health. The medical profession can give notional assent to the need for prevention of disease and promotion of health but often justifies the undue proportion of ever-diminishing budgets spent on treatment by speaking of 'public demand'. The pattern of high spending on drugs as a major priority for a country's health plan as well as for individual families in their struggle for health has serious consequences for both the economy and the well-being of people in Europe but in poorer countries the results can be devastating. Sanders (1985) gives the example of Tanzania – as he says, certainly not an extreme example – of the consequences of this perspective: the projected drug bill for 1980/81 of the Ministry of Health was 40 per cent of the national health budget. On the micro-level, poor, underfed people, suffering from diseases of poverty and a general situation of marginalisation, frequently believe that they have to spend what little money they have on drugs in an often desperate effort to keep their families alive. Any health worker who feels inclined to blame a poor Latin American, African or Asian mother for ignorance when she spends her last coins on vitamins or on an incomplete dose of antibiotics rather than on food for her malnourished child would be better advised to look at the experiences of health and health care which have formed the mother's judgement. And if blame is to be laid at anyone's door, it should not be at that of the mother but at the door of those who exploit her poverty for their own profit. Neither can we pass by the door of those health workers who are happy to leave intact and unchallenged the medical model of health care with its emphasis on drugs because their interests are served by the existing situation; to challenge and seek to change it might call for an enormous effort, if not heroism: the road facing anyone questioning the medical model and its alliances with the pharmaceutical profession is not only not very rewarding, it can be dangerous.

In our search for what role pharmaceuticals should play within a whole health care system, one would do well to remember the words of Medawar: 'Among the main causes of serious ill-health are poor nutrition ... lack of effective preventive measures and care – and mainly in developing countries, lack of clean water and sanitation as well' (Medawar, 1984: 13).

To suggest that the dominant medical model is an engineering one which puts too much emphasis on institutions such as hospitals and on pharmaceuticals is not to deny the importance of either of these components in a rational health policy, it is simply to point out the distortions and even suffering which can occur when they are given undue importance. Drugs 'do "play an important part in protecting, maintaining and restoring health", but only when used well' (*ibid*, quoting WHO: 13).

WHO's examination of the role of hospital services in a rational health programme has involved a serious look at the existing unhealthy relationship between hospitals and the pharmaceutical industry. A background briefing paper for a conference on the role of hospitals in PHC says that a teaching hospital should be in a symbiotic relationship with the health needs of the community it is supposed to serve. In other words, the health needs of the general population should determine the priorities and professional preoccupations of the teaching hospital. Unfortunately, according to the WHO study this is very rarely the case. Rather, these hospitals are in symbiotic relationships with 'the industry which has produced the scientific and technological base on which the teaching hospital now rests' (Paine and Siem Tjam, 1988: 19).

Technical solutions to social problems

The health-care model, then, which non-Western countries have sought to emulate for all kinds of understandable reasons is a model which is hospital-based treatment and pharmaceutical dependent and centred on the deployment of expensive doctors trained at considerable cost as medical engineers. This model dominates the allocation of health resources in these countries as it does also in the West. Professor Banerji, in India, has been a coherent and consistent voice exposing the folly of following the West along the road mapped out by the medical model. He records that in his own country rationality tried to assert itself and in an effort to critically assess the development of its health services the Government of India asked itself whether it had done the right thing in adopting a model of medical services and health care which was more expensive than India could afford and which emphasised curative rather than preventive and promotional dimensions of health care. Banerji quotes the Indian Government in its 1982 National Health Policy which laments the mismatch between health needs and service provision brought about by following too closely the guidelines of the Western model: 'The existing situation has been largely engendered by the almost wholesale adoption of health manpower development policies and establishment of curative centres based on the Western models, which are inappropriate and irrelevant to the real needs of our people and the socio-economic conditions obtaining in the country' (Government of India, Banerji, 1985: 32). But as Banerji says, the questions have been asked in India but not as yet properly answered.

One of the ironies of this imitation and sometimes imposition of Western health care, of the Western model on the cultures of developing countries is that, as we have said in Chapter One, what is being copied or promoted is a truncated version of the Western health care model. Western health care systems have to be understood as having a history. The current admittedly curative and medical-intervention focus of present health care systems in Western societies stands on the historic basis of the whole powerful public health era and its achievements which have already been mentioned. It is widely recognised that high morbidity and mortality from infectious diseases were reduced in Europe through public health interventions like the provision of clean drinking water and the safe disposal of human waste. 'Wonder drugs' had little to do with this process (McKeown, 1976). Curative care and individual medical interventions are like the branches of the tree of which the roots are these great public health activities. This, alas, is not considered when Western health care systems are exported: the branches and fruit are taken and the roots which are not in 'medical' science are forgotten. Atrophy is inevitable.

Meanwhile, the focus on inward circles is still seen to be the essence of scientific medical practice and a pledge of progress and the ultimate conquest of disease. In the early 1990s a cyclone devastated parts of Bangladesh and cholera, which is pandemic in the country anyhow, was the inevitable result. Almost at the same time cholera spread through many countries of South America, where it had been thought of as under control, long since. The medical world rejoiced in the development of preventive measures. Public health? Improved living conditions? Investment in anti-flooding public works, surely, in the case of Bangladesh, to limit the disease? No, to all of these. The rejoicing was in what was reported as the successful development of a vaccine against the disease of cholera. A medical, technical solution is the presumed answer. This is almost a caricature of the medical model and a distortion of a health care system founded on a solid base of public health; it is also far from the vision of a health system proposed at Alma Ata which would combine curative, preventive and educational dimensions. What we are left with is a technical-curative system which sees prevention almost exclusively in terms of vaccines, a medical rather than a health system.

The international crisis concerning the Acquired Immune Deficiency Syndrome (AIDS) and the response of the medical services provide us with another example of the narrow technical focus of the medical model. There is wide acknowledgement that, faced with such an incurable viral complaint, the engineering model of health care is at a loss and the only hope lies in education and prevention. Nevertheless, the major spending is not on these, but on research to discover a vaccine (Macdonald, 1990). As we will see in Chapter Eight, even when emphasis is put on AIDS 'education', the influence of the medical model often encourages an undue emphasis on medical technical information and 'patient compliance'. With some few exceptions this makes for very unsuccessful AIDS education.

The limited vision of health and health care encouraged by western medical systems has led to a distortion of many health programmes, including PHC programmes, as we shall have occasion to point out in the next chapter. Sometimes the wider circles of causality of ill-health are acknowledged – poverty, poor housing etc. – but the tackling of problems in these dimensions is put on the shoulders of the community itself or of some underpaid community-health worker.

It is, of course, in the interests of the medical profession as it currently sees itself to continue to base its work on a model of health care which is based on the manipulation of high technology; ill-health as a 'technical', rather than a social-political and economic problem. As we saw in the last chapter, in the early 1990s Bangladesh has witnessed the curious situation of doctors denouncing health reforms which would have helped provide a more rational and equitable health service. Of course, if one accepts the dominance of the medical model and its alliances with a certain distribution of resources, this support is not so curious.

Efforts to widen the model

There have, of course, been calls for several decades for a wider vision of health and ill-health. Some of the most notable calls for a wider paradigm have come from the discipline of mental health. The limitations of the vision of health work fostered by the engineering model manifest themselves in the world of mental health care in a particularly striking fashion. A very large proportion of the conditions presenting to general practitioners and family doctors in Western countries are connected with mental health and psychological stress; more and more, the gap between such need and clinical training is being acknowledged (McWhinney, 1983). The proper functioning or harmony of bodily functions is only part of human health and well-being and is intimately bound up with psychological harmony and well-being. The study and treatment of stress, for example, is forcing a more holistic view of human health on medical practitioners as greater insights are gained on such matters as the complex interplay between the body's immune system and such non-biological factors as social support and sense of self-worth (Research Unit in Health and Behavioural Change, 1989).

An important paper from George Engel based on the experience of psychiatry made a deservedly well-known appeal for a vision of health care based on a 'biopsychosocial model' (Engel, 1977). There is some criticism of Engel's approach for not really offering a step towards a new paradigm despite the rhetoric (Armstrong, 1987). But there can be little serious doubt that the call for a biopsychosocial model represents an important questioning of the medical engineering model as the inadequacies of this are felt in the world of mental health. The comparison of the human psyche to a machine and the disturbed psyche to a broken-down machine does not provide the most useful framework or terms of reference for the person charged with the complicated process of 'repair'. Engel draws his example from schizophrenia; in the management of this condition and in others there is a growing acceptance of the important interplay between what we have come to think of as 'mind' and 'body'. Evidence shows that, although theoretically the medical world acknowledges this interaction, when front-line doctors are faced with the complications of psychosomatic illness they often are unable to decide what to do. A study in the UK showed differences in general practitioners' willingness to take decisions about the diagnosis and treatment of a considerable number of conditions where a neat separation of causality or specific aetiology was not possible and where the lines between *soma* and *psyche* are blurred:

> Medical education teaches undergraduates about the diagnosis and treatment of known diseases or illnesses. In general practice, very few problems presented by patients are so neatly diagnosed. They may present with problems at a very early and undifferentiated stage, or they may present with a combination of many social, psychological and physical ills that are difficult, if not impossible to unravel (Bucks et al. 1990: 546–7).

It is difficult not to see that the roots of this unease of physicians lie in the medical model of health which still underlies most medical training: 'Physics, chemistry and biology are considered to be the sciences basic to medicine; ... the question therefore, is not whether the engineering approach is predominant in medicine, which would hardly be disputed, but whether it is seriously deficient as a conceptualisation of the problems of human health' (McKeown, 1976: 6).

Even when there has been a concerted effort to widen the circles of medical concern, to attempt to bring more of an emphasis on health rather than simply on disease, as in the approach laid out by the Canadian Government in its White Paper of 1974, *A New Perspective on the Health of Canadians*, the inbuilt bias towards the individual and the bio-physical has a tendency to influence actual policy. This, at least, is the finding of Evans and Stoddart (1990): the Canadian White Paper proposed that the determinants of health status could be categorised under the headings of *lifestyle, environment, human biology* and *health care organisation*. It presented a broad view of health and health care, encompassing what we have called outer as well as inner circles of causality and thus seemed to call for a series of actions including social interventions to improve the health status of citizens. However, this message was filtered through a medicalised interpretation with the result that it came to mean 'that people are largely responsible for their own health status – have in fact chosen it'. The focus became individualised and medicalised. An emphasis on healthy eating which, for example, in the original document would have seemed to imply public as well as individual actions, actually led to interventions focusing more narrowly on the individual. The policy emphasis came to be on high serum cholesterol, resulting in a sharp increase of people on drug therapy and regular monitoring, a clear medicalisation of a public health message. Consequently, the 'behaviour of large and powerful organisations, or the effects of economic and social policies, public and private, were not brought under scrutiny'. The conservative force of the medical vision is very strong indeed and is often, as in this case, wittingly or otherwise, in tandem with other conservative forces in society. We are witnessing many examples worldwide of the focus on the individual's responsibility to improve his/her health. This is clearly a political agenda since it turns attention away from the social construction of ill-health. The medical model is a powerful ally of forces which resist improvements in the social fabric of society. With another understanding of health, a wider perspective of the causality of disease, the medical profession could be a formidable force for change.

Some commentators from within the medical profession, using the framework of ideas supplied by Kuhn, have noted the beginnings of what can be called a shift in the medical paradigm. McWhinney, for one, from the world of family practitioners in North America, charts what he sees as the emergence of a new paradigm in medicine (McWhinney, 1983). He sees the conventional medical paradigm as having served us well; but, rooted as it is in nineteenth century science, it suffers from the limitations of its origins and needs to change to incorporate our increased understanding of the human condition. Based on a system of 'differential diagnosis', (in a perspective of specific aetiology), the work of the medical profession is to prescribe a specific remedy or ameliorating intervention. This approach works well, says McWhinney, where a single intervention like an antibiotic or surgery can alter the prognosis. But it does not fit for many of the illnesses which family practitioners have to deal with. Linked to this, the distinction between mind and body often limits the medical vision. McWhinney suggests that this situation of mismatch between need and medical vision is leading towards the emergence of a new paradigm which will 'pay more attention to health' and oblige medical practitioners to be more than technologists. In the world of international health it could be said that it has been the experience of mismatch between problems and existing 'solutions' which has given rise to initiatives like the PHC approach.

Even at its best, when it does have a prevention and educational 'arm', the medical model tends to allocate these activities to peripheral or more marginalised colleagues: sanitarians or 'health assistants' or, in the West, to Public Health doctors or 'Health Promotion' officers. The medicalisation of public health has been noted (Research Unit for Health Education, 1989) and it is interesting to record that in Britain in the early 1990s many Departments of Community or Public Health felt the need to change their names and call themselves departments of 'Public Health *Medicine*', perhaps in an effort to hold on to their medical credibility. Surely Public Health should rather be holding on to a vision of health care where medicine has a role alongside prevention, rehabilitation and promotion but is not the all-important factor. A major effect of the dominance of the engineering model of health care has been that prevention and education are not considered to be part of the main-stream health activity and have constantly to be 'medicalised' in order to be respectable. 'Health' has come to mean 'medicine' and, as shall be argued, Primary Health Care has come to be equated with primary medical care. In this way its challenge is diluted and ultimately lost sight of altogether.

The Alma Ata Declaration of Primary Health Care has a degree of freshness, some would say innocence or naïvety, about its language and its optimism. As we have said, there has been a certain amount of support, or at least tolerance for the comprehensive approach proposed by Alma Ata as long as the focus of its attention was the countries of the Third World. But the model of health care which it seeks to displace is the model of health care which is dominant in most societies, not only in non-industrialised ones. If it poses a challenge, it is to established policies and practice of health care everywhere. It deserves a closer look.

Chapter Three

The What of Primary
Health Care: Alma Ata

In the broad lines of the Primary Health Care approach as laid out
at the Alma Ata Conference in 1978 it is possible to see the
framework of a new health care model with universal significance.
Primary Health Care is presented by the Conference as a health
system integrated into the development plans and programmes of
a nation: 'It forms an integral part both of the country's health
system, of which it is the *central function and main focus*, and of
the overall social and economic *development* of the community'
(WHO, 1978: VI, emphasis added).

It is unlikely that the countries which signed the document in
1978 realised the full significance of what they were endorsing. It
will take still more years before we realise the full significance of
what it means to make PHC the 'central function and main focus'
of a health system and the consequences of this for daily practice.
Many Third World countries have tried to take this definition of
PHC seriously; it is surely a valid question to ask those health
workers in Western societies who feel that they are involved in
primary health care: do they think that they understand PHC as
at least potentially forming the 'central function and main focus' of
their health systems? Is it not rather some fairly minor activities
to do with the periphery of the health services?

Moreover, it is very useful and important to have the links
between 'development' and health and, consequently, between
'underdevelopment' and ill-health, brought to our attention in
such a straightforward manner as in the above words of Alma Ata.
Health workers, according to the PHC approach, are development
workers and development workers can also be health workers.

Thanks to the issues raised by the PHC approach, it is
increasingly difficult for any health planner, especially in a
country which has the principles of PHC written into its national

health policy, to plan a *medical* service rather than a *health* service. Of course, there is no real dichotomy: health care must always include medical care. But in the twentieth century there have been (and in many circumstances still are) distortions and contradictions which have resulted in an over-emphasis on the role of medical technology focused on the treatment and possible cure of disease to the neglect of wider strategies of health-promoting and prevention activities. Health care has often meant medical care and sometimes even very limited medical care. Such an emphasis has become less and less tenable since the Conference of Alma Ata, one of the greatest contributions of which was to call into question the medicalisation of health. The Conference had a focus on the countries of Asia, Latin America and Africa. But there is a recognisable similarity between health or medical services all over the world. In Chapter Two we have seen that there is an international medical culture: a cluster of attitudes, policies and practice that we can describe as the medical model. The PHC approach which has emerged in the third quarter of the twentieth century challenges this model and questions some of its assumptions and the policies which flow from it. Once such questioning has gone on in one part of the world, it is valid and even necessary to ask if similar questions should not be raised elsewhere, in this instance, in the industrialised countries which exported the model to the Third World in the first place. Alma Ata has raised the issues, asked the questions. It is possible that medical historians or health service historians of the future will ascribe considerable importance to Alma Ata. In the conference document we can detect the first clear signs of policies which not only challenge the medical model, well entrenched since the beginning of the twentieth century, but which also present the first outlines of a new health care model. The Trojan horse of PHC is inside the walls of the medical fortress. It is important to remember that it is often to the so-called developing world that the industrialised world must turn for examples of the new model in practice. It is in the non-Western countries that the medical model has been most exposed for its inadequacies and where PHC approaches have begun to emerge. As the flaws in the conventional medical model become clearer in Western societies as well, these can learn from the countries of Africa, Asia and Latin America where it is possible to find some examples of the emergence of a more dynamic, rational and holistic health care model.

Of course, as we have said, Primary Health Care includes primary medical care. But is not synonymous with it. The vision of health care enshrined in the Alma Ata Conference stresses the promotion of health and the prevention of disease, but it includes, of course, the treatment of conditions of ill-health: 'PHC addresses the main health problems in the community, providing promotive, preventive, curative and rehabilitative services' (Alma Ata Declaration, VI 2). Central to PHC is the balance between different aspects of health care. The approach builds on the successes of the existing medical model, but at the same time confronts its weaknesses as well as the imbalances which it has brought and sets out to provide an alternative way of conceptualising and planning health services.

Much of what is described in this chapter in terms of ideas and practice and which, using the vocabulary of the Alma Ata Conference, we will call the Primary Health Care approach, exists under other names in a whole variety of contexts. This is a point to which we will have to return. For the moment, it is enough to say that the broad outlines of the PHC approach can be identified in many health policies and significant numbers of current health care programmes in Latin America, Africa and Asia. These policies and programmes have their origins, directly or indirectly, in the Conference of Alma Ata and represent an emerging alternative paradigm of health care.

In the European context, there has been a parallel development which also owes some of its inspiration to the Conference of Alma Ata. This has been called the Community Health Movement and also challenges the medical model, presenting another way of dealing with health and health services, stressing collective action to promote health and people's partnership with health professionals to this end (Jones, 1990). The initiatives which can be described as belonging to this movement are, as Jones points out, often efforts to tackle inequalities in health and take a Community Development approach to health care. It is surely useful to recognise this movement as part of the global PHC effort. Experiences in both societies would be of mutual value if the links were recognised and encouraged.

In the Third World context, one can trace the growing discontent concerning the limitations of health services to debates and experiences in the 1960s and 1970s. The debate was crystallised in the Conference of Alma Ata in 1978 and in the preparatory meetings which led up to it. This preparation consisted largely of a reflection on the efforts of countries and health programmes to work towards a health service which would more adequately address the health needs of their populations. This often involved initiatives which went beyond the limitations imposed by inherited structures and health policies with their strong emphasis on treatment and cure and underemphasis on such matters as health promotion and the prevention of disease. One hundred and thirty four countries were signatories to the declaration of Alma Ata and its ideas and vocabulary have passed into the policy and planning documents of many of these, and other, countries since that time. Critics will say that the ideas have gone no further than the policy documents which contain them. This may be true in some cases, but what will be argued here is that the PHC model of health care poses such a challenge to the medical model that it is inevitable that resistance will be encountered when attempts are made to put it into practice on any significant scale. Nevertheless, in terms of the history of ideas and of medical institutions, the ideas of Alma Ata and PHC are relatively new. Several decades constitute a short time for an alternative approach to make policy inroads on such a powerfully entrenched system of thought and action as that represented by the conventional medical approach.

The document of Alma Ata is the result of an international conference and this itself lays it open to certain sorts of criticism: it tends to be normative, saying what should be done rather than how to go about doing it. But it has to be said that many of the documents which WHO have published subsequently represent efforts to further elaborate what the practice of PHC should be. Some critics say that the changes Alma Ata envisages will not come about without changes in the larger fabric of society: for example, it argues for a fairer health system and it is a well-rehearsed argument that we will not have a fairer health system unless we have a fairer society (Navarro, 1982). This matter will be dealt with at greater length when we deal with the equity dimension of PHC where it will be suggested that health workers concerned with a more just health care system cannot postpone all action aimed at reforming the health services while waiting for the radical social transformation which would bring a better world.

Some health practitioners are now familiar with the concepts and ideas of Alma Ata without realising the origins of that vocabulary: 'health for all', as we shall see, is a slogan currently widely used in health campaigns. Often those who use it do not realise that it has its origins in Alma Ata and in that context is much more than a campaign slogan. 'Participation' (or 'community involvement in health' as some now would have it) and 'intersectoral collaboration', key ideas of Alma Ata, are also used (or misused) frequently. They are referred to either with enthusiastic approval or with considerable contempt, without those using them realising that they form essential pillars of the PHC approach and sometimes without there being too much in the way of understanding of the meaning and consequences of these ideas.

The meaning of Primary Health Care

PHC is often understood in terms of campaigns or programmes within medical services or to mean health projects run by non-government agencies on the periphery of the medical system. This is not the meaning of PHC as put forward by Alma Ata. The conference envisaged PHC as a radical reinterpretation of health services. For the conference, 'health for all' represented a commitment to greater justice and equity in health-resource allocation; this involves a denunciation of existing inequalities and, at least implicitly, the resolve to redress such imbalances. This commitment to equity is one of the essential pillars of the PHC approach. Another is the adherence to the principle of the right of people to be involved in significant decisions concerning their health services, the participation dimension of PHC, now increasingly referred to as community involvement in health, CIH. The third pillar of the PHC philosophy is the acceptance of the need for the medical profession to collaborate with other sectors which make significant contributions to the health of populations. This is referred to as intersectoral collaboration. These three 'developments' as Tarimo and Creese (1990) call them, are the basis of the PHC approach. They represent an enormous challenge to medical thinking and practice. Until Alma Ata, these three dimensions have been severely underdiscussed in the health sector; now they are on the international health agenda and are, at least, more difficult to ignore than they have been in the past. They represent both the ideals of a new approach and a major challenge to existing policies and practice. The medical world can dispute the usefulness, the appropriateness, the feasibility of the PHC approach, but these three pillars erected by the Conference demand an examination of issues that cannot easily be dismissed.

As we have said, the content of the Alma Ata Declaration and the policies it endorses are much discussed in the Third World. But in Western societies it must be said that Alma Ata is not as well known as it deserves to be. Research in 1983 and 1985 shows that those responsible for the teaching of doctors for general practice and public health, both in the UK and in Europe, show a remarkable ignorance of Alma Ata, and, so presumably, of its contents and challenge (Walton, HJ, 1983, 1985).

There is a 'definition' of Primary Health Care in the Declaration of Alma Ata. It is a definition which has resurfaced repeatedly in health-policy documents throughout the world. Although there is an overall consistency, the text bears all the marks of a composite authorship, probably the result of Conference members' discussions and the attempt to incorporate their differing experiences. It is clear that every form of writing belongs to a literary genre of some kind, determined largely by its contextual origin and its purpose, and this is also true of the Alma Ata Declaration. It would be inappropriate to reproach the author of a report of a football match in a newspaper for not treating the topic as would an anthropologist in an academic journal. The definition of PHC in Alma Ata has to be understood in the context of the literary genre of international conferences, marked inevitably by the rhetoric of United Nations 'speak'. This in itself does not diminish the validity of its ideals. The definition is to be found in Section VII of the Declaration:

> Primary health care is essential health care based on practical, scientifically sound and socially acceptable methods and technology made universally accessible to individuals and families in the community through their full participation and at a cost that the community and country can afford in the spirit of self-reliance and determination (Declaration of Alma Ata: VI).

This is as dense a definition as any that one is likely to meet: it combines the idea of the best in technical medicine coming to meet the health needs of communities in as culturally appropriate and inexpensive a way as possible and seeking some kind of partnership with communities in the maintenance of health and tackling of disease. It holds up an ideal for health-care providers. Many countries in the Third World have tried to make the definition come alive and put it into practice. Real attempts at partnership between professionals and communities abound in these countries. They are much less common in Western societies where the medical model is more deeply entrenched. Many health-care teams in Latin America, Asia and Africa would not be shy to test their own practice against such a yardstick; it would also be an interesting exercise for any health team in industrialised countries.

In order to show the usefulness and the application of the

definition, we will apply it here to a programme of traditional birth attendants (TBAs), meaning the PHC initiative which initiates collaboration with traditional midwives in order to improve birthing practice. Such programmes are now common in many communities of the developing countries. As applied to TBAs, this part of the Declaration can help us envisage what might be a PHC approach to an appropriate health service concerned with birth: TBAs should be trained in 'practical' and 'scientifically sound' methods and technology. This is generally not problematic: when conventionally-formed midwives and gynaecologists are involved in sharing their knowledge at the community level, we can expect that much of their focus will be on hygienic practices which are scientifically sound and practical. But the introduced methods and practices must also be as 'socially acceptable' as possible: the PHC worker must be not just a provider of a service, but someone working in tune with the cultural norms of the community. In the context of TBAs, this would mean the acceptance by the health professional of such cultural practices as peer support for the mother and a variety of birthing positions other than the supine position when these others are the cultural norm. The PHC definition suggests some kind of partnership: the professional working with persons in the community who preserve traditional beliefs and practice. In the context of birthing practices, the community 'partners' are clearly the group of women we know of as TBAs (it is obvious that where such a traditional cadre does not exist, PHC programmes would try to apply PHC principles in some other manner and not necessarily try to artificially create one).

This scientific and socially acceptable technology should also be made 'universally accessible' to individuals and families through their full participation and at an affordable cost. If we apply this to the example of TBAs, we would be looking to these TBAs to bring support to all mothers in any community, especially those of modest means and living at some distance from institutions of health care, generally underserved by conventional Western medicine. TBAs help to realise the PHC aim of access to health care for all. 'Participation', 'self-help' and 'self-determination' must also be involved, according to the definition. The partnership with the community which is part of the PHC approach must be one which accords the community partners an active role. In our example, the TBAs would not be the 'lackeys' of the health service (Werner, 1982), but members of the community whose work is esteemed and enhanced through contact with the health services.

The definition also mentions affordable costs at both country and community level. PHC programmes should involve rational costing throughout the whole of a national health care system. In the case of birth practice, this must mean a balance between equipping the tertiary hospitals' maternity wards with appropriate technology and allocating sufficient resources for the training and support of those responsible for assisting at births at the community level as well as for the funding of referral cases by TBAs of expectant mothers with conditions whose management they are trained to recognise as lying outside their competence.

The definition continues by situating PHC within a wider context:

> It (PHC) forms an integral part both of the country's health system, of which it is the central function and main focus, and the overall social and economic development of the community. It is the first level of contact of individuals, the family and community with the national health system bringing health care as close as possible to where people live and work, and constitutes the first element of a continuing health care process (*idem*).

We have a vision here of PHC which does not allow it to be marginalised and considered as only some activities at the periphery: PHC involves a directing of the national health services to community health needs. Unfortunately, as we have seen in the previous chapters, national health services have rarely been planned according to such a rational assessment of the community's needs and appropriate solutions. PHC also involves a conscious effort to see health as an integral part of the nation's development; health planning and development planning must go together. As regards the example of TBAs, the consequences of these dimensions of the PHC approach would be that their work be respected as an important part of national health policies concerning childbirth. TBAs would not be ignored by the modern system but would be in partnership with it. This part of the definition says that PHC involves the interface between people's health needs and the health service, suggesting some level of health-care worker accessible to everyone. Sometimes this part of the definition is seen in isolation from the rest and PHC is said to consist only of the first level of contact between people and services. It is clear from the rest of the definition, however, that a much wider concept of PHC is involved. Its activities must be 'part of a continuing health care process'; the TBAs we are speaking of must be linked to higher levels of care both by support and guidance and as part of a referral system: the knowledge that she is supported and valued and that she can refer her clients to more sophisticated levels of care is essential to the community-level worker.

In the European and North American context the PHC approach might not lead to the development of partnership between TBAs and health professionals, though the medicalisation of birth is a topic worth examining. But for the purpose of illustration, it might be useful to look at what could be described as a PHC initiative in Ireland. In Dublin the Community Mothers' Programme demonstrates several of the principles of PHC. Young mothers in the community are supported by Community Mothers, volunteer workers from the community who are supported by Family Nurses (Johnston, in print).

Secondary and tertiary health care cannot be said to be part of 'Primary Health Care' but they must be part of a health-care system which is turned towards the needs of the community in the spirit of PHC. All must be integrated into a rational entity. This is the spirit of the Declaration of Alma Ata; it deserves a further look on account of the perspectives it offers on an alternative approach to health services.

Access to health care

Much of what health care is offered to the majority of the populations of the Third World and poorer segments of Western society as well is often inaccessible. The curative hospital-based model of health care is, almost invariably, urban-biased and so, almost by definition, access is denied to many people. Even physical proximity, however, does not mean facility of access, since economic constraints also bar many from the use of such institutions of health. The lack of access is a mark of the health services in many countries. Primary Health Care comes to challenge such a situation: 'PHC is essential health care ... made universally accessible ... at a cost the community and the country can afford and is the first level of contact of individuals, the family and community with the national health system, bringing health care as close as possible to where people live and work' (VI).

As we have said, PHC is not, of course, only the basic level of health care; it involves a reorientation of the whole system to support people's health needs, with a real flow of communication and support through the system: '... it should be sustained by ... referral systems, leading to the progressive improvement of comprehensive care for all' (VII). Seen in this perspective, 'health for all' is more than a slogan, a pointer towards some ideal future, it is a denunciation of the fact that many people are often denied access to health care, since it acknowledges that at present we have only 'health for some' or 'health for the few'. 'Health for all', when adopted by a health service, is therefore a commitment to greater access for as many as possible.

Cultural appropriateness of health services

The Western model of health care in the Third World was, in terms of the values it perpetuated, part of a country's colonial inheritance and therefore often inappropriate for local needs. It also promoted attitudes of disdain towards local health resources. Cultural invasion, the process whereby an indigenous people are encouraged to consider their cultural values as inferior, has made a huge impact in the area of health. PHC, as proclaimed by Alma Ata, demands of all involved in the health service a reappraisal of this situation. Local needs should be at the heart of the health services and local perceptions, wisdom and experiences should be valued: 'PHC reflects and evolves from the economic conditions and socio-cultural and political characteristics of the country and its communities ... and relies also on the collaboration of traditional practitioners' (VII).

This is a far cry from the denunciation of traditional healers as 'witchdoctors', which is how many such traditional healers were often described by Western health workers. More dangerously, it was how many indigenous health workers recruited to work in Western-type medical services in their own country were trained to speak about traditional healers in their own societies. The legacy lingers. Seeking the collaboration of traditional healers calls for an enormous turn-about in attitude on the part of all such health workers. Conceptually, however, the call for such collaboration is simply the corollary of the famous definition of health by WHO as the complete psychological and physical well-being of individuals and communities. The PHC approach takes the definition seriously and starts from the position that we build on the resources for health and healing which already exist in individuals, families and communities. This approach is clearly hampered by the history of the alliance between the arrogance of Western medicine and supposed colonial superiority which dominated the establishment of health services in Third World countries.

Health-centred health services

In the form that Western health services developed in the Third World there has been a very strong emphasis on institutions, on those who staff them and on the treatment dispensed in them; prevention of disease and promotion of health have been given considerably less emphasis, or are seen to be peripheral to the real business of health care. PHC confronts this imbalance and sets out to address 'the main health problems in the community, providing promotive, preventive, curative and rehabilitative services accordingly' (VII). Of course, these are only the declared aims of a document. The gap between rhetoric and reality can be very wide. But the stated aims of Alma Ata highlight existing distortions and increasingly oblige health workers and planners to take a position on the issues they raise. In this case, the conventional, often unchallenged, position has been to accept the high proportion of slender national health budgets being used to provide machinery and personnel whose focus is not prevention or promotion but treatment of disease. The PHC approach acknowledges the importance of curative care but sees it as being necessarily linked to 'promotive, preventive and rehabilitative services'.

Prevention

In theoretical debate, prevention is acknowledged as being important in conventional Western medicine: 'prevention is better than cure', but in fact, the overwhelming focus of health services is on treatment. As we have seen, the health services are often reactive, rather than proactive; the medical model on which these services are based has been called the 'fire-engine' model of health: the firemen do a good job, but their main task is to wait until a fire has started and then attempt to put it out. Even when medical services attempt to adopt a strategy of prevention, the medical model encourages an often almost exclusive focus on interventions such as immunisation: there is a tendency to imagine that if we can vaccinate a community against disease then we have done the major preventive work that is called for. This may be true in a perspective of primary medical care but it certainly does not fit with the philosophy of Primary Health Care promoted by Alma Ata. Vaccination is a technical intervention delivered by the health profession to a hopefully receptive community; as a form of 'prevention', it fits well into the notion of the 'solution' to a given problem consisting of a technical medical 'fix'. There is no doubt of the importance of vaccination campaigns but they cannot possibly represent a health system's entire responsibilities in the matter of prevention.

A vaccine-centred prevention approach is limited. In the first place, there is no vaccine against many conditions. AIDS gives us a tragic example of the limitations of the medical model's narrow focus on treatment/vaccination. Reason tells us that prevention must be a major plank of any anti-AIDS policy. The rhetoric of the medical world acknowledges that education is the only vaccine for AIDS that we are likely to have for some considerable time (Sabatier, 1989; Macdonald, 1990). But the whole medical system is geared to treatment and to cure. Both of these at the moment are beyond our reach but vast sums of money are spent on them, money that could be used for education, the only *real* vaccine against the condition. The present orientation of the medical system and the training of the medical profession does not allow for any genuine commitment to such a 'vaccine'.

A commitment to prevention would involve a much greater emphasis in medical training on health and ill-health in society, on what we have called the outer circles of causality. Factors in the environment which enhance or detract from community health would be a necessary focus of study and professional preoccupation rather than the present almost exclusive concern with individual pathology. Ayurvedic medicine, the traditional health system of India, takes for granted that medical workers are interested in and study the nutritional, life-enhancing properties of food. It proceeds on the rational assumption that human well-being depends to some extent at least on the quality of what we eat. Health enhancement and prevention of disease are a major preoccupation. The virtual neglect of the study of nutrition in most Western medical schools shows just how far we are from such an approach.

Passive or active responses? The challenge of participation

Western scientific medicine puts the doctor in a central active role in health care and encourages an attitude of passivity from patients and communities. The word 'patient' itself conjures up the idea of docile receptivity. Alma Ata, on the other hand, asserts that 'PHC requires and promotes maximum community and individual self-reliance and participation in the planning,

organisation and control of primary health care and relies on ...
health workers including physicians, nurses, midwives ... and
community workers ... as well as traditional practitioners ... to
work as a health team' (VII). Doctors trained and socialised in
Western allopathic medicine have some readjustments to make in
their professional attitudes when called upon to take part in team
work and when asked to encourage active participation, rather
than passive acceptance, in their clients. Carlaw (1988) talks of
the 'shifting role of the health professional for Primary Health
Care'. In his overview of examples of PHC practice in Africa he
points out that community-based PHC such as called for by Alma
Ata calls for a partnership between health professionals and the
community, which he sees calling for 'a vast change in relationships and authority'. Participation is one of the key demands of
PHC. By specifying that this participation must be in 'planning,
organisation, operation and control of primary health care', Alma
Ata is distancing itself from the practice of participation consisting
of 'patient compliance', a form of participation the medical world
does not find threatening or controversial. The expression itself,
'patient compliance', indicates the kind of partnership foreseen by
the medical model: the public carrying out the prescriptions of the
medical profession. As we will explore further in Chapter Five,
Alma Ata endorses the more rare form of participation, in
decision-making and evaluation; this gives people a much more
active role in the promotion of health and management of disease
and can sometimes be perceived as a threat by those formed in
more conventional forms of health care. This present chapter sets
out the broad outlines of the PHC approach and some of the
challenges it poses: notable among these is people's participation
in health care. Consequently, the meaning and implications of
community involvement in health and the consequences of this
dimension of PHC for health professionals both deserve fuller
treatment and are addressed in later chapters.

From microscope to macroscope

In conventional health-care, the regular focus of concern is, as we
have said, individual pathology. Alma Ata takes a wider view,
which incorporates a concern for the treatment of individual
symptoms but acknowledges that problems of ill-health can have
structural causes, causes which lie outside the control of an
individual and even sometimes outside the control of whole
communities or countries. Alma Ata states clearly that injustice

is at the root of many problems of disease. The Conference lamented this situation: 'The existing gross inequality in health status of the people particularly between developed and developing countries as well as within countries is politically, socially and economically unacceptable' (Declaration of Alma Ata: V).

Primary Health Care, as envisaged by Alma Ata, is part of human development and involves a commitment to equity from both people and governments, which have 'a responsibility for the health of their people which can be fulfilled by the provision of adequate health and social measures ... in the spirit of social justice' (*idem*).

There is a tendency in health-care services to deal with ill-health as though it were a technical problem. As we have argued, problems of poverty tend to be understood by the health profession in medical terms, they tend to become medicalised, and so the proposed solutions tend to be medicalised as well. The vision of PHC is that the health worker's vision must expand, to include wider circles of disease causality. There must be a move away from the vision encouraged by the microscope to one provided by what we have called the 'macroscope'. The wider circles of disease causality must be part of the professional health perspective. As one researcher said of the wider socio-economic and political factors: 'The nature of the local and world contexts ... appears clearly as generating more and more social inequalities which have severe consequences in terms of health' (Fassin, 1991: 25). To give a stark example: nutrition programmes in the perspective of a narrow medical model pay considerable attention to vitamin and nutritional supplements, to the techniques of growth monitoring and health education programmes which instruct mothers on the basic technical knowledge of a 'balanced diet'. The perspective is on 'inner circles', on the biological and on individual lifestyle and behaviour, well away from the socio-economic condition of the family, its purchasing power, even its access to land on which to grow food and, of course, well away from international structural adjustment problems (the 'outer circles'). The PHC approach addresses these issues; not, of course, by pretending to solve them, but by situating the individual or community which is suffering within this wider context; not blaming people for their ill-health, not pretending that good health is always within the control of people's actions. This necessarily means a readiness to work with all other agencies which promote improved quality of life for the community. It is not hard to see how a narrow medical perspective fits with a status quo in which inequalities are rife and which does not want any inspection at all of the social and economic causes of poverty and ill-health.

The 'microscopic' view is not, obviously, limited to health workers in the Third World. Its contradictions are simply more evident there. We can find examples of it in all societies. In Glasgow, Scotland, for example, it took tenants of a housing association many years to prove what they already knew: that a considerable amount of ill-health, especially in the child population, was due to the unhealthy environment in which they lived. Scientific studies were used by them to illustrate this (Martin *et al*, 1987). A macroscopic view of ill-health was called for from health workers, a view that would include the wider circles of health and disease causality and not focus only on the treatment of symptoms. The Easterhall Tenants' Association had such a view, such a wisdom, but no one else had.

The more doctors and other health workers, as well as aid agencies and charities keep their vision of the problems of ill-health in a medical perspective which concentrates on symptoms and individual pathologies, the less likely they are to run into trouble from defenders of the status quo. The broad view of health and ill-health and its causes which is adopted by Alma Ata would seem destined to run into opposition coming from several quarters, not least of all certain sections of the medical profession. This opposition has indeed been voiced and shows the strength of the challenge posed by PHC.

The PHC approach as declared at Alma Ata has a more holistic view of the nature and causes of health and disease than is encouraged by the standard medical view. This perspective builds on WHO's much quoted, sometimes derided, definition of health as 'a state of complete physical, mental and social well-being, and not merely the absence of disease or infirmity' and this is further elaborated upon by Alma Ata. Health is 'a social goal whose realisation requires the action of many other social and economic sectors in addition to the health sector (I) ... PHC includes ... at least education, ... nutrition, ... safe water and basic sanitation, ... maternal and child care, ... immunisation treatment ... and essential drugs' (VII).

So, from the declaration of Alma Ata, we see something of a reaction to a narrow medical approach to health care and the emerging characteristics of an alternative approach. Central to PHC understood in this way is the commitment to a more just distribution of health resources. Health care is a right, not a favour or a more or less affordable commodity. Central also, is the demand for people's participation and the consequent need for the medical profession to relinquish some of its power in the matter of health care. Linked to this is the demand for a holistic view of health as part of human social development which obliges health workers to acknowledge the contribution of other sectors: this is the demand for an intersectoral approach.

PHC has its 'component parts', some of which are listed in the document. Such programmes, like MCH (Mother and Child Health), nutrition programmes and community health-worker schemes must be seen, in the spirit of Alma Ata, not as the characterising marks of the approach, since they exist in many forms elsewhere, but as programmes which have to be inspired by the PHC philosophy. All of these component parts or 'essential elements' can be transmitted in a way which is top-down, non-participatory and far from the spirit of PHC, or they can be infused with the demands of justice, participation and an intersectoral approach. Programmes would have the same name in the two approaches but will be radically different in their professional practice and in the impact on the community. The failure of 'selective' PHC (programmes which target one or more of the elements of PHC) to significantly reduce overall mortality rates (Kasongo Project Team, 1981; Economist, 1986) does not point to the failure of PHC but to the failure of health services to implement a *comprehensive* PHC approach along the guidelines laid down in Alma Ata. As we will see in Chapter Four, it is much less demanding for health service workers to add an 'element' or two of the list of components of PHC to their existing programmes and to engage in selective versions of it than to face the challenge of a comprehensive PHC approach which tries to take seriously the equity, intersectoral and participation dimensions of the original vision of Alma Ata (Newell, 1988).

There are those who say, for reasons that are understandable, that the name 'Primary Health Care' should be dropped since we are overloading such a title if we want to include the above listed ideals. Some insist that we should speak of 'community health' or 'community-based health-care' or 'participatory health care', rather than Primary Health Care. The great problem about these different alternative names for PHC is that they *are* different from one another; by refusing a common name to initiatives and programmes which have the same characteristics of the approach spelled out by Alma Ata, we can actually undermine the struggle for an alternative approach to health services and dilute the impact of Alma Ata. The medical establishment can more readily adjust to, and even incorporate, a variety of 'programmes' in different parts of the world: programmes of 'community health' in India, of 'community-based health care' in parts of Africa, programmes of 'health for all' in cities in Europe. Many of these programmes in fact represent what Alma Ata calls a Primary Health Care approach. Giving the manifestations of the approach different names does not totally disempower the initiatives but it can diminish their collective impact. The search for more correct or accurate titles and the refusal of the common name, 'Primary Health Care', removes the positive advantage of a shared banner.

It has to be acknowledged that although the rhetoric of PHC is now widely apparent in many national health policy documents, it is less common to see it in practice. This gap between the words and the deeds has led some to dismiss PHC altogether. A little too quickly, perhaps. Most serious commentators acknowledge the need for further clarification of the concept of PHC and certainly for some examination of both its rationale and the obstacles in the way of its implementation.

It is not everyone, by any means, who is ready to write off the challenges of PHC as being irrelevant. There are those who, while acknowledging the importance of wider social change in the improvement of the health of communities, would argue the case that in Alma Ata we have an important milestone in the move towards a new medical paradigm or model. Certainly, people involved in PHC programmes often find themselves going 'beyond the clinic', not only in terms of a move beyond the constraints of health institutions and an extension of work into the community, but also in the matter of attitudes, with health professionals in PHC finding themselves going beyond the parameters assumed by their initial clinical training. It has been said that the medical paradigm is under pressure to change and the pressure, as is often the case in the shift in paradigms, comes from the margins of the discipline in question; in the case of medicine this pressure has come from such areas as the discipline of psychiatry (McWhinney, 1983). But the pressure for change has also come from the move towards PHC in developing countries, from such trends as the community health movement already mentioned and from the experiences of community development and adult education throughout the world.

It is not only the countries of the Third World which have adopted the principles of Primary Health Care as expressed at Alma Ata. The WHO Regional Committee for Europe in 1984 set itself some important targets for health care in the years leading up to the twentieth century. Target 26 of these states: 'By 1990, all Member States, through effective community representation, should have developed health care systems that are based on primary health care and supported by secondary and tertiary care as outlined at the Alma Ata Conference (WHO, 1985: 99). This being the case, it is clearly important that WHO member states increase their understanding of what Alma Ata meant by Primary Health Care. It is important that the concept and its application to policy be clear. Virtually all countries throughout the world have elements of the PHC approach adopted into their national health policies. The challenge presented by the PHC approach is considerable. In Third World countries, the challenge was so great that almost as soon as the approach was declared and programmes to implement it were launched, opposition to it became institutionalised. 'Selective' PHC was born, a weaker and, it will be argued, a 'medicalised' version of the real thing. This is the focus of the next chapter.

Chapter Four

The Selective Option: The Medicalisation of Primary Health Care

One of the most important international debates on the matter of new approaches to health services has to do with the choice between what has come to be known as *selective* Primary Health Care and *comprehensive* Primary Health Care. This is not an arid academic discussion about terminology or philosophy. The debate concerning selective/comprehensive PHC can and does lead to crucial policy decisions being made which have a considerable impact on the form health services actually take, especially on the choice of who is to be served. The position taken by policy makers on this matter affects the quality of life of millions of people. The debate concerning selective or comprehensive PHC and the policy positions which result can also be seen as offering us an illustration of the response of medicine to the challenges of the PHC approach.

In the light of what has been said already about Primary Health Care and the medical model, the selective version of PHC can be understood as a medical view of PHC or a medicalisation of the original PHC message. Given the medical model, and the way it has shaped health services in many countries, one could have predicted that comprehensive PHC as put forward by Alma Ata would tend to find itself subsumed into a medical view of the world and have its impact and challenge inevitably diluted. This is just what has happened in many quarters. It is one thing for the holistic principles of PHC to be clearly spelled out in Alma Ata and for these principles to be endorsed in national health programmes: participation, working with other sectors in the development of communities, equity. The policies are there, but they are often implemented by health services and medically trained practitioners already cast in the mould of medical care, the medical intervention model. The pouring of PHC principles into such a mould often has the effect of diluting the impact; PHC becomes medicalised. There is an inbuilt tendency in systems informed by the medical model to reduce health interventions to medicotechnical interventions and to reduce the role of people's participation in health, essential to the initial vision of PHC, to something that looks suspiciously like collective patient compliance. This medicalisation of PHC is an aspect of the debate about the choice between selective and comprehensive versions of PHC which is often overlooked. Awareness of this tendency to medicalise and so undermine the PHC approach could go some way towards resisting this bias and so preserve some of the real force and impact of the comprehensive vision of PHC presented at Alma Ata.

Selective PHC has been called 'weak' PHC and comprehensive PHC 'strong' (Wisner, 1988). The approach of PHC as presented by Alma Ata (the strong version), has a radical edge, posing a challenge to existing medical thinking and practice. This it does by insisting on the need to go beyond a medico-technical approach to ill-health; the macroscopic vision of health and ill-health sees health-enhancing actions outside medicine as its legitimate concern. Comprehensive PHC indicates that approach concerned with health 'for all' and in addition understands health as part of development. This necessitates on the part of health workers a wide, long-term and holistic view of both the causes of ill-health and strategies to be followed to promote health. Comprehensive PHC sees collaboration with other sectors and people's participation in the search for solutions as essential components of PHC under the overall umbrella of a movement towards greater equity in health care.

Alma Ata, without any doubt, presented a strong version of PHC, a comprehensive view, insisting on the role of sectors such as agriculture, water and sanitation and education; it is the task of health workers to collaborate with these sectors since they make a major contribution to health and an appropriate health care system along PHC lines must be operationalised as part of 'the overall social and economic development of the community'. The documents which have followed the Conference have continued to stress this collaboration (see, for example, WHO, 1979; 1986; 1988). The comprehensive approach presented at Alma Ata gave considerable importance to people's involvement in the health-planning process; participation, in this view, is not an optional luxury but a crucial dimension of health services. An editorial in *Tropical Doctor* goes so far as to say that the choice is now between health care *delivered* to populations or participatory health care, which sees the involvement of the community as being essential for effective health programmes (Lankester, 1991).

Likewise, the comprehensive approach brings the matter of justice and equity on to the discussion table in health matters and into the planning process: health workers and programmes which try to implement a comprehensive approach find themselves being called upon to acknowledge the poverty and material deprivation dimension of disease; this often brings PHC supporters to be involved in anti-poverty programmes and in people's struggle for a more just distribution of resources. An international group of PHC workers was discussing the major health problems in their respective countries. Asked to identify the major cause of ill-health, they gave answers such as malnutrition, people's ignorance etc. Then came the turn of a woman from Kerala in India, a member of a people's movement: the major cause of ill-health, she said, was injustice (Macdonald, 1987). The woman from Kerala was speaking from experience. The collective reflection and action of the group she belonged to had sharpened her perception. Alma Ata denounced the 'gross inequalities' in health status between countries and between sections within countries, thereby committing PHC not only to be conscious of such disparities but to be involved also in the struggle to remove them. With this vision of social reality, PHC workers are sympathetic to, if not directly involved in, the struggle of people with their social, economic and political environment in the building of a context which promotes their health.

Promoters of selective PHC, on the other hand, what Wisner calls the 'weak' version, while applauding the aims of comprehensive PHC, argue that, since time and resources are limited, health workers must select and target for intervention those conditions of ill-health which are most amenable to low-cost technology. This line of thinking leads to such conclusions as those of the Bellagio Conference called by the Rockefeller Foundation to discuss this very matter: 'until comprehensive primary health care (CPHC) can be made available to all, effective services aimed at the few most important diseases (selective primary health care – SPHC) may be the best means of improving the health of the greatest number of people' (Warren, 1988: 891).

Some researchers draw our attention to the political dimensions of the move from 'strong' to 'weak' versions (Banerji, 1984), suggesting that programmes with targeted interventions characterised by 'appropriate' technico-medical interventions to be delivered to the public by health workers can help to obscure the need for political and social reform to remove structural barriers to health. Many health workers are not responsible for the overall approach of the systems or programmes in which they work and sometimes are too involved in the day-to-day tasks of programmes to realise some of the more general implications of the priority decisions made in these programmes. International agencies have had considerable influence in determining the focus of much health work in developing countries with the financial and 'moral' influence they bring. These agencies are often very interested in selective PHC and have been the main proponents and funders of this approach. Comprehensive PHC has long-term developmental goals with aims sometimes as general as the 'increase in people's confidence in their ability to control some parts of their environment'. This can be unattractive to agencies who have an in-built need for short-term achievable goals: they want to contribute to improved health but need to be seen to be so contributing. Long-term development strategies stressing participation are not very glamorous and are in pursuit of goals which are not easy to measure. The promotion of participation and equity as strategies for achieving improved health status are often seen by the health profession as secondary or even disposable dimensions of health-care projects; they also have little place in a conventional view of dealing with disease.

Moreover, it is obvious that the equity dimension of PHC can be embarrassing to international agencies; by adopting the medico-technical view of 'selective' PHC they can involve themselves in initiatives which tackle ill-health, or at least its symptoms, without challenging any of the underlying social causes of disease. Some commentators show the links between the West's economic recipes for Third World countries, especially 'structural adjustment' policies and the promotion of social initiatives which do not challenge the status quo: the encouragement of selective rather than comprehensive PHC is a good example (Kanji 1989). As often, there is here a close fit between a medical view of disease and symptom-focused interventions and the interests of those who at present profit from the status quo. It is important for health workers in the field to realise that some seemingly praiseworthy health programmes stressing the short-term technical interventions of selective PHC can be serving the interest of those who are positively against the sort of social change that a move towards comprehensive care would call for. The arguments are rarely spelled out in this fashion. Selective PHC, when it is promoted, is always put forward as being the most rational option for health intervention, the most 'feasible' and the one most appropriate to medical workers.

No sooner had the Conference of Alma Ata finished and its policies and philosophy or approach been brought to international attention and indeed begun to find their way into national health documents than the scope of PHC as proposed by the Conference began to be whittled down and its challenge eroded. There was little criticism of the aims of PHC as presented by Alma Ata: health for all through increased popular participation and intersectoral collaboration. But some voices were raised immediately (as soon as one year after the conference) to say that these aims were too idealistic and that there was a need to be selective, to target conditions of ill-health which could be perceptibly and cost-effectively improved upon. We cannot do everything all at once, it was argued, so let us choose what can reasonably be tackled. Let us target those most at risk, specific diseases with high morbidity and mortality and amenable to non-costly interventions. The focus should be on health technologies which can have the greatest impact at the lowest cost. Moreover, some proponents of this approach argue that many poorer countries lack the 'institutional capability' to implement a comprehensive PHC approach. In situations of 'problems of scarcity and choice', 'the strategy to improve health must be selective. Success will depend heavily on correctly identifying the most important problems in each population group, selecting the most cost-effective interventions, and managing the services efficiently' (Warren, 1988: 892).

There are those who suggest that the distinction between selective and comprehensive is an artificial one and that in practice all health programmes are necessarily selective, since they all involve some form of prioritisation; no programme can tackle all problems at once and so selective PHC, it is argued, can be seen as the first step towards comprehensive PHC. Of course, some health programmes begin with certain limited interventions and build up to more comprehensive coverage. But there is a difference in a comprehensive health plan which sets out to meet the health needs of 'all' through strategies beginning with some groups and those selective programmes which target high-impact interventions to the exclusion of entire groups of people with chronic conditions. There *is* a difference between the two approaches and perhaps the acid test is to ask: does a programme plan to move towards access for as many of the population as possible? Is there some form of genuine community involvement? Is there any effort to work with other sectors? In other words, are there any signs of the 'three pillars' of PHC in the programme or does it remain a medico-technical intervention, primary *medical* care? Any programme which avoids the 'three pillars' of PHC and has some outreach programme of a particular service should realise that that is what they have, an outreach programme, an extension of health services, not PHC. Other voices warned that selective PHC was not PHC at all and as a strategy it risked to undermine the very principles of PHC. Newell says that the seeds of the selective approach lay in the lists of suggested 'elements' presented at the conference. Although Alma Ata stressed the *process* of PHC in the way we have described in Chapter Three, it put forward possible elements of PHC programmes. These were often leaped upon as being PHC: simple curative care, monitoring of nutritional status, immunisation programmes etc. As Newell says, the danger is that when you start with any list, 'the entire reasoning starts to change and the list becomes the objective' (Newell, 1988: 904). In fact it is entirely possible to have health-care programmes with some and even all of the 'elements of PHC' but delivered to the community in the conventional top-town manner by health professionals. Such interventions should not be called PHC at all. To give them this name is to rob PHC of all its impact and challenge. The selection of one or other of the elements of PHC as an area for activities which will be conducive to measurable impact can allow health professionals to drop the imperative to work with other sectors, or in partnership with people and to put off indefinitely the equity dimension of PHC. Behind the debate about whether selective or comprehensive is the most appropriate strategy there lies, in fact, the struggle for the survival of PHC as an alternative approach. Selective PHC is no threat or particular challenge to anyone; it suits the style and objectives of many donor agencies and fits well into the engineering model of health care.

The case for selective PHC has probably never been better put than by its first protagonists, Walsh and Warren, in 1979, the year after Alma Ata: 'Until primary health care can be made available to all, services targeted to the few most important diseases may be the most effective means of improving the health of the greatest number of people. The crucial point is how to measure the effectiveness of medical interventions' (Walsh and Warren, 1979: 152).

The heart of the selective approach is the proposition that it is both practically and morally incumbent on us to look for the means which allow us to have the greatest measurable impact at the lowest cost and in as short a time as possible. The arguments put forward by Walsh and Warren in favour of a selective approach to PHC have been used in justification of many programmes which target particular diseases or age groups. The ideals of comprehensive PHC, the argument goes, are fine and praiseworthy, but in the harsh world of reality we have to accept that some diseases and conditions of ill-health are not amenable to simple technical solutions. We cannot afford, in terms of either time or money, or both, to be comprehensive. By implication, though this is never spelled out, the elderly and chronically ill must be put aside for the time being, indefinitely, in fact. Measurable change will come about through the targeting of infectious diseases of childhood. So let us make an impact where and how we can. Examples are programmes which target diarrhoea or measles in children. Often such programmes are called PHC though, as we have said, there is little place within them for the 'essential developments' of PHC, namely, concern for equity, participation and intersectoral collaboration. Primary Health Care becomes a package which can be delivered by health professionals to individuals in the community. It is significant that Walsh and Warren talk in terms of 'services being made available': strong PHC is not just concerned with services being made available, but with people's involvement in determining the nature and scope of such services; it is not 'delivered PHC' it is rather 'participatory PHC' (Lankester, 1991).

The researchers Walsh and Warren also speak of the importance of measuring 'the effectiveness of medical interventions': this way of thinking seems to equate health care with medical care and there is little scope in this vision of health care for other dimensions of health-related activities like those connected with education and agriculture, or with social support for the elderly or chronically ill. As has been said, instead of a multisectoral approach aimed at the root cause of inequalities in health, we are presented with a package of technical interventions or 'fixes' like growth-monitoring or oral rehydration (Farrant, 1989). Selective Primary Health Care might more accurately be called primary medical care. In this view of things, PHC becomes, not a people-centred empowering process, but a mere extension of certain low-cost existing medical services. This can be seen as a predictable reaction of those formed in what we have described as the medical model to ensure that PHC remains within their own parameters of influence. The medical model tends to reduce health care to a series of packages to be delivered, after diagnosis, by a doctor, or someone who looks as much like a doctor as possible, to the individual patient, the 'receiver' of health care. In community programmes, the receiver/patient is the community itself. Once the problem has been 'diagnosed' (and this is often done without consulting the community at all; the profession decides what is wrong) the prescription follows: a CDD (Control of Diarrhoeal Disease) programme or an ARI (Acute Respiratory Infections) programme, or some such already-packaged intervention. Under the name of PHC one or more technico-medical interventions are decided upon and implemented by the health services. Of course, the collaboration of other sectors and the involvement of the community are desirable objectives but not absolutely necessary. All this is a travesty of PHC as proposed by Alma Ata.

One of the clearest voices raised against selective PHC is that of Professor Debabar Banerji. He says of the selective PHC approach, 'This movement not only tends to fragment a health care system and takes it away from a wider ecological, intersectoral and integrated approach, but it also actively hinders community self-reliance and seriously erodes the democratic rights of the people to participate in decisions which so vitally concern them' (Banerji, 1986: 231). Professor Banerji sees selective PHC as a solution conceived of by Western agencies which overlooks indigenous experience of countries and the epidemiological evidence built up over time of the interlinking between diseases and the need to tackle them comprehensively (Banerji, 1984). He condemns the attempts by the West to impose what he sees as untested and epidemiologically unsound approaches on non-Western countries. Previous vertical programmes like the campaign against malaria have failed and this failure has shown the need for a broad integrated approach which acknowledges the links between diseases and the need for intersectoral collaboration. Alma Ata called for such an approach, yet all this has been set aside very quickly by the proponents of selective versions of PHC, what Chen calls 'derivatives' of PHC (Chen, 1988). Selective PHC seems, on one level of argument, both reasonable and manageable, perhaps especially when the planners are at some distance from the people who suffer from the synergistic links between diseases and between disease and poverty that we have described. Most importantly, selective PHC does not call for any significant shift of resources, nor indeed for any transfer of power. It is a non-threatening version of PHC and one easily contained within the existing status quo.

UNICEF has been prominent in the promotion of selective PHC in the form of its programme called 'The Child Survival Development Revolution' ('revolution', interestingly, has been dropped in some countries which adopted the programme because the word had unpalatable connotations). In its UNICEF form, PHC becomes GOBI and GOBI-FFF: a series of 'simple, cost-effective solutions to major problems'. G is for growth monitoring, O for oral rehydration, B for breastfeeding, I for immunisation, FFF for food supplements, female education and family planning. In later years water and sanitation have been added by some programmes. Many health workers find in this simple formula a manageable and effective interpretation of PHC. Manageable it may be, but in what sense can it be said to be effective?

As we have seen, poverty and a web of socio-economic conditions linked to it are at the root of many health problems in poor communities. Can we make a significant difference to the health status of communities by focusing on individual diseases, through selective PHC? It is perfectly understandable that the medical profession would be drawn to such an approach, in the light of what has been said already about the medical model and its predictable search for a technico-medical solution to health problems. With its doctrine of specific aetiology, allopathic medicine seeks to knock out the causative agent of particular diseases in the body: a pill for every ill. Therefore there is a predisposing favourable attitude to the 'simple technical solutions' of selective Primary Health Care as strategies for dealing with the enormous health problems of poor countries. Huge efforts have been put into the targeting of one disease at a time. Smallpox eradication seemed a great success and such targeting a model to follow. Unfortunately, the targeting of other individual diseases like malaria has proved very unsuccessful and should have warned us against selective approaches. As an example of the failure of the selective approach to tackle one disease, Franco-Agudelo cites the example of the Rockefeller Foundation's anti-malarial programme in Latin America which adopted a technico-medical approach to the disease. The exclusion of the social determinants of ill-health from this programme made sure that the health programme was removed from any call for structural change in the spirit of social justice. The medical model fitted well with this approach. All the efforts against the disease focused first on the fields of biology and physiology, and then on chemistry and chemotherapy. At the same time, all possible social determinants were relegated to a secondary, barely scientific role. In other words, this meant the rise of the individual-biology aspects' preponderance at the expense of socio-structural ones (Franco-Agudelo, 1983: 61).

The failure of anti-malarial programmes has to be acknowledged. Malaria is even on the increase in many countries. As has been said, this should have alerted health service providers to the flaws inherent in selective technico-medical approaches. Unfortunately, the medical model is alive and well and its appeal in PHC continues in the selective versions of PHC which governments and the medical profession feel drawn to.

Another striking argument in favour of thinking and planning in terms of comprehensive rather than selective PHC comes from the work of the Kasongo Project Team in Zaire in their measles-eradication campaign reported in the Lancet (The Kasongo Project Team, 1981). Measles was targeted and successfully eradicated in an entire district of around 200,000 people. This would seem like a success story in terms of selective PHC; the logic presumably being, now we have successfully knocked out one disease (measles) let us target another. The impact on health status seemed to be good, since morbidity figures and measles-related mortality figures improved. If the research team had stopped its investigations after a few years, big conclusions might have been drawn about the success of selective PHC. Fortunately, the approach was more scientific and continued to look at impact on mortality rates over time. It was found that the targeted intervention had only a short-term impact on overall mortality figures. As the team themselves reports, for the targeted group of children, 'survival probability ... tended to diminish afterwards, to approach that of the unvaccinated group'. In other words, although the targeting of one disease was 'successful', in terms of removing the condition (measles), it was not successful in terms of improving the overall life chances of the children involved. After a relatively short time the children who had not died of measles died of some other infection, doubtless, like measles, linked to malnutrition and certainly the underlying poverty of the communities involved. Selective, targeted programmes are seductive both to aid agencies, anxious for short-term observable 'results' and to the medical profession in its search for technical solutions to disease. It is surely not too strong to say in this context that such efforts, with short-term clinical 'success' and 'coverage' but often negligible long-term impact on the reservoir of poverty-linked diseases, could be better described as activities of primary medical care rather than primary health care.

The above example shows that targeted groups, even though helped at one stage of their lives, can – and in the context of poverty will – suffer at a later stage when the conditions which cause the ill-health are not addressed. Moreover, in selective Primary Health Care, what can be said about the chronic conditions? What about the health of the elderly and the well-being of disabled people? 'Health for all' must be replaced as a slogan, it seems. Selective PHC can be seen as an attempt to alleviate some of the worst consequences of failing to provide a comprehensive health care system. The basic 'demands' of PHC are almost totally removed: equity, people's participation and intersectoral collaboration get shelved. As a WHO document, overviewing the period since Alma Ata, says, 'the selective approach fits the technological and political orientation of some donor agencies who look for concrete objectives and measurable outcomes, achieved in a relatively short period of time; in embracing these characteristics of selective programmes, they might ride roughshod over fundamental principles of community-based PHC' (WHO, 1988: 44).

The use made by some programmes of Oral Rehydration Therapy (ORT) offers us another good example of the dimensions of selective Primary Health Care. Oral Rehydration Therapy (ORT) has been hailed as one of the most significant medical breakthroughs of the twentieth century. Instead of trying to treat diarrhoea, a great killer of children, with ineffective antibiotics or expensive and elusive intravenous fluid (IV) therapy, it has been discovered that the condition can be effectively treated with oral administration of a saline/carbohydrate solution, often sugar and salt in water. We have noted that those who promote the comprehensive version of PHC are in no way denying the importance of 'elements' of PHC such as the control of infectious diseases like diarrhoea: rather, they would see the necessity of situating this sometimes very important part of PHC within the wider context of the improvement of the social and economic environment in which most diarrhoeal disease takes place. The 'comprehensivists' are not all academics: I was being shown around a section of the town of Dhaka in Bangladesh by some health workers who were part of a large DD (diarrhoeal disease) campaign. They were anxious to show the extent to which social marketing of ORT had had a beneficial influence on the public. I was led to a family house and after introductions the topic of DD and ORT was raised. The atmosphere suddenly became charged, with the grandfather of the house gesticulating excitedly and leading me by the hand out of the door and round to the backyard with the ORT workers in tow. He pointed to the water pumps, the source of water supply for several families. The pumps were submerged in foul water. The man continued his explanation and the ORT workers were somewhat shamefacedly obliged to tell me what was being said (and in fact had no need of translation): the whole family knew how to make up a home-based oral rehydration solution and they used it frequently in the home. But the cause of the problem remained the water supply and it was with that that they needed help. The social marketing of the 'appropriate' technology, the medico-technical intervention of oral rehydration was addressing the symptoms of the problem and ignoring the cause. I remember the incident as an example of local wisdom and common sense evaluating service-provision. The elderly man was also making an eloquent case for comprehensive as opposed to selective PHC. ORT has a real but limited usefulness and only as part of a more comprehensive solution to the problems of diarrhoeal disease.

One of the most respected people in the area of appropriate health care for disadvantaged communities must be David Werner, author of such important books as *Where There is No Doctor* and *Helping Health Workers Learn* (Werner 1978, 1982). Werner himself has done much to promote oral rehydration and yet he insists that it is a 'stop-gap measure' which supposes that the intervention is part of a wider programme of tackling the causes of the disease (Werner, 1988).

The result of some empirical research in the Caribbean and in Bangladesh corroborates this questioning of ORT in vertical, selective programmes and sees these as being 'unlikely to reduce mortality due to diarrhoea substantially unless the dysentry-malnutrition syndrome is tackled at the same time'. The same study goes further and, about ORT programmes, concludes that 'efforts to reduce malnutrition in countries such as Bangladesh could be better directed to ensure that the poor have more access to food' (Fitzroy Henry et al, 1990: 4 and 5). The flaws of the arguments in favour of selective PHC could not have been exposed more tellingly; *food* and not *ORT* is often the appropriate health response. ORT is only one example of the seductive but dangerous attraction of selective interventions. Quick technical fixes such as promoted by some practitioners of 'PHC' are far away from the spirit and approach proposed at Alma Ata. As Farrant has put it: 'The effect of this promotion of SPHC under the PHC umbrella is to keep health interventions firmly within medical control and to detract from the need for long-term social, economic and political change' (Farrant, 1989: 8).

In such a perspective, the attempts to persuade us that the choice between selective and comprehensive versions of PHC is an artificial one (Mosley, 1988) remain largely unconvincing. Rifkin and Walt have argued that the promotion of selective PHC is a departure from the key principles of PHC (Rifkin and Walt, 1986). The late Professor Ken Newell argued that the difference between the two versions is a real one which it is important to grasp since the choice of one or the other approach has far-reaching consequences. The support of international agencies for selective PHC has direct and indirect influence on the choices made in health planning in many countries. Such choices are 'the national expressions of technical SPHC (selective PHC) decisions tied to international or bilateral resources in New York, London, Geneva or elsewhere and are signs that the battle is not just ideological but is one which will have its ultimate expression in villages and homes' (Newell, K, 1988: 905).

A meeting in the Netherlands in 1985 described the selective approach as a 'problem-by-problem' approach as opposed to the 'multi-causal' or comprehensive approach and denounced the selective approach as a 'dangerous technical illusion' which diluted the impact of the PHC challenge (de Bethune et al, 1985; Grodos, B. et al, 1988). It remains to be seen whether the seemingly strong arguments against selective PHC will win the day and change policy. There are many obstacles to the adoption of comprehensive PHC and not least of these are the inbuilt tendencies of the medical model of health care.

The three pillars of genuine PHC, participation, intersectoral collaboration and equity, have been mentioned at several points in the discussions so far; separately they will form the topic of the next three chapters.

Chapter Five

The First Pillar: Participation

There is much talk of participation in programmes of health care which claim to follow the philosophy of PHC and/or 'Health for All'. For some years we have been told by WHO that 'community involvement in health' (CIH) is the preferable expression. Whether we choose to speak of participation or community involvement in health, in either case it is clear that what is meant is, at the very least, a more active role for the beneficiaries of health programmes. This suggests that conventional health-care systems expect a generally passive role from such beneficiaries, a point that has been illustrated in Chapter Three when describing the consequences of the medical model. The term 'participation' has now become commonplace and is so often used by health planners, health workers and international health organisations that they sometimes give the impression of having invented the whole notion. Far from it. The idea of people participating in programmes has some considerable history in the world of development; health professionals now interested in the notion should be ready to learn from this accumulated experience.

This chapter will take a brief look at the history of the promotion of people's participation in the field of development work and how the word has been understood in order to see what lessons there might be for those interested in participation in health programmes. The problems inherent in the promotion of participation within the medical model will be looked at in more detail. Finally, we will describe the move towards greater participation of populations and individuals in health care, including through the PHC movement, as well as considering briefly the need for structures to mediate any participation.

Participation in development

The vocabulary of 'development', in the way it is now frequently used by governments and international agencies, only became common currency in the 1950s and 60s as former colonies and former colonisers after World War II adjusted to the changes this war had brought and set about planning for the future. In these two decades there was the strong belief that development meant economic growth and modernisation along Western lines. It was accepted that, as a country modernised, initially only a few people would profit, but the benefits would ultimately 'trickle down' to the less-advantaged. The economist Rostow was very influential in this matter; he described the 'five stages of growth' which all countries would need to follow if 'economic take-off' and modernisation (i.e. development) was to be achieved (Rostow, 1960). The ultimate goal of 'developing' countries would be to come as close as possible to the patterns of development of industrialised countries. The theorists of rural development – for this development was principally seen as concerning agricultural workers or 'peasants' – developed a sociology of rural development, much of it with a view to understanding the resistance to change by these peasants to the diffusion of innovations of development. The major obstacles in the way of this development were seen to be the backward attitudes of those 'least developed' which led them to resist change and a major task of the developer was to understand and remove such barriers (Rogers, E, 1969). The Green Revolution was perhaps the supreme example of this sort of development, understood as the introduction of innovations: new farming technology was introduced including new hybrid seeds, with the aim of providing food for the developing world. More food was produced but too often by the few for the benefit of the few (Mehmet, 1978). Doyal sums up the reasons for this failure, with words which should ring a warning for all health workers: 'The main reason clearly lies in the fact that the green revolution proclaimed the possibility of a technical solution to what are in fact socio-economic problems' (Doyal, 1979: 130).

With the perceived failure of this paradigm – basically, benefits did not 'trickle down' and development eluded the majority – the development model was challenged and a new one looked for (Macdonald, 1981). About this time, in the 1970s, a whole host of thinkers, especially from Latin America, were denouncing the dominant theories of development as being pernicious (Frank, 1967). Instead of looking at development as some benign process of growth from 'underdeveloped' to 'developed', it was argued that it is more useful, accurate and insightful to place the process in an historical perspective; before we can speak of 'development', we should analyse the process of underdevelopment and the creation of dependency, powerlessness and marginalisation. We should understand the 'development of underdevelopment'. One application of this analysis to Africa resulted in the forthright book of Rodney, *How Europe Underdeveloped Africa* (Rodney, 1972). The basic contention of this and other such works is that if we wish to make sense of the development process and the challenges it faces, we have to come to terms with the many years of exploitation and underdevelopment which developing countries and communities within them have suffered (Macdonald, 1986). Relevant to the discussion of people's participation is the notion of marginalisation: instead of benefits of development reaching all the population, large sections of the population in Third World countries became marginalised, pushed away from any active role in deciding the shape of society or often their own lives. In an analysis of the development process in Latin America, O'Sullivan-Ryan speaks of this marginalisation in terms of 'non-participation': 'marginality is a situation of non-participation for certain groups of the population, a situation that is begun by an economic system incapable of offering permanent productive employment to those groups and that extends itself to the other spheres of social life' (O'Sullivan Ryan, 1980: 77). (Although O'Sullivan Ryan is talking here of Latin America in the 1970s, it is remarkable how relevant his vocabulary is to contemporary industrialised countries where 'marginality' and non-participation are also common features of the society and where promised benefits of development are still not 'trickling-down'.)

Anyone interested in 'educating' populations in the processes of participation must be ready to face the reality that many people have been educated in a long school of marginalisation, non-participation. There are those who point out that the peasant resistance to change, far from being a sign of backwardness or 'fecklessness', represented a very rational response to what was unknown, and unproven (O'Sullivan, 1980). What was happening in the late 1960s and 1970s was that the simple equation of development with economic growth was being challenged. From a variety of ideological positions a vocabulary of 'people-centred development' and 'people's participation' began to emerge. At first it was seen as a useful means to an end; behind the concern for increased people's participation in development was sometimes an understanding of people as 'human resources'. As the United States began to expand its influence on 'developing countries', its policy of participation in development was spelled out, both in terms of what was meant by participation and why it was deemed to be a necessary strategy for these societies. Title IX of the United States Government's Foreign Assistance Act states that it had become 'increasingly clear that the failure to engage all of the available human resources in the task of development not only acts as a brake on economic growth but also does little to cure the basic causes of social and political instability which pose a constant threat to the gains being achieved on economic fronts' (in Cohen and Uphoff, 1980).

The economic undertones of this statement are clear, as is the implication that participation is expected to promote political stability. Participation makes good economic sense and promotes the political and social stability necessary for development. Participation, in this light, is clearly a means to an end, an 'engine' of development, a process to be encouraged to maximise the modernisation of a country and to preclude the possibility of social unrest. The Brandt Commission's Report of 1980 was very much in this line when it spoke of a growing consensus around the idea that egalitarian reforms and increased participation by all sections of the populations of the Third World is able to substantially improve conditions for more rapid and stable growth (Brandt, 1980). Development in this light is seen basically as a transfer of technology; the requisite participation by people was adoption of the new technology (Cohen and Uphoff, 1980).

But there were also those who saw participation in the process of development, not just as a means to an end, of achieving some goal, but an end in itself, a goal worth pursuing on account of its intrinsic value. Participation was seen as a 'good thing' and not just a means to an end but a value worth pursuing in its own right. One way or another, participation became one of the key words, if not *the* key word in development circles in the 1970s. As the 'trickle-down' theory of development was denounced, organisations like the International Labour Office (ILO) began promoting a development strategy to meet people's basic needs. Development was not to be equated with economic growth alone; social development was also very important and participation was seen to be a key element in the process. A logical progression from the idea of people-centred development is the idea of people-generated development: the community not just as the recipient of development but as the principal actor in the process:

participation is itself a basic need of the people, and it must be included as a critical consideration in any development strategy ... It is through action generated by one's thinking and initiatives that men and women give expression to their creative facilities and develop them and thereby develop further as human personalities. It is for this reason that participation is a basic human need (ILO, 1978: 1).

The interest in development circles in participation led not only to the inclusion of the term in most development policies but to some attempts to clarify what is meant by the concept and to examine what is actually involved when an attempt is made to promote strategies of participation in practice. Of particular importance here is the work of a group of researchers from Cornell University in the United States under the leadership of John Cohen and Norman Uphoff. With the financial backing of USAID, this team of researchers set about analysing development programmes which claimed to be participatory. The resulting reflections (Cohen and Uphoff, 1977, 1979, 1980) remain very useful documents for all parties interested in people's participation in any social programme.

Although the analysis of Cohen and Uphoff is quite sophisticated, the basic insights are not complicated. They set out, they said, to 'seek clarity through specificity': by being specific about what kind of participation was involved they hoped to bring greater understanding to the rather vague notion of participation. They developed a taxonomy of kinds of participation based on what they had found in their research. The four most important kinds of participation they identified were: participation in implementation, in benefits, in evaluation and decision-making. The distinction is a simple one; one can argue about whether evaluation is not really just a sort of decision-making, and so perhaps these two kinds of participation should be dealt with together, but that does nothing to diminish the usefulness of their taxonomy for analysis. The simple framework can be a powerful tool in most circumstances where participation is spoken of but the actual process remains not so clear. If one asks oneself, which of these kinds of participation is referred to and actually takes place, many ambiguities fall away.

Participation in implementation was the most common kind witnessed by the Cornell researchers: people are often asked to join in and offer some kind of contribution to a programme, most often through their labour, though sometimes through financial contribution or offerings in kind. This indeed is one kind of participation and is often what is referred to in health projects as participation, involving people in, for example, carrying bricks, or in contributing in some other material or financial way to programmes set up to benefit them. This participation in benefits was also quite commonly noticed by the Cornell researchers: if a well was dug, or a school or dispensary built, some of the people at least benefited from the product; in that sense they 'participated'. Again, it is to be hoped that many people participate in the benefits of health programmes executed on their behalf by governments and health agencies.

Cohen and Uphoff found the other kinds of participation: in decision-making and evaluation, to be at once the least common but perhaps the most significant kinds of participation. These are the important kinds of participation, since through these processes people have the opportunity to become 'owners' of what is going on rather than remaining in the role of mere recipients of programmes which others have designed for them. The researchers note that these kinds of participation (in evaluation and decision-making) are rather rare in social programmes. As has been said, it is possible to see evaluation and decision-making as being linked: evaluation is a form of decision-making: the evaluator decides on the value of something that has taken place. One might say that Cohen and Uphoff force us to see that the core of real participation lies in decision-making. Look for this kind, they say; there you will see whether there is any genuine participation.

Other researchers, notably in ILO and UNRISD (ILO, 1978; UNRISD, 1979), carried the process of clarification of the meaning of participation further by stating (what may seem to be the obvious) that implicit in involvement of people in decision-making, and evaluation of what is done in the name of their development, is the acknowledgement that participation is about power.

The people whom we are calling upon to participate are often those individuals and sections of the community previously denied the power of decision-making in development; they can be thought of as having known non-participation. In terms of power, they are the people who have suffered what we have called 'marginalisation'. The thinkers of the 'development of underdevelopment' (or dependency) school of thought that have been mentioned already help us to understand how individuals and communities and indeed whole nations can be caught in a trap of dependency. This analysis helps shift the focus from supposed 'deficiencies' of individuals, cultures and nations as accepted causes of under-development and helps us look for explanations in the structural powerlessness they have experienced over many generations: 'The deficiency view of the causes of underdevelopment has been challenged, if not discredited, by new analyses. The analyses link the conditions of underdevelopment to a history of unequal power relationships between the Third World and technologically advanced countries from the era of colonialism to the present' (Kindervatter, 1979: 18).

The powerlessness referred to here is not only of Third World countries faced with the dominant power of the West, it is equally the powerlessness of marginalised sectors within these countries and, ultimately, of the least privileged individuals. The relation-ship between poverty and powerlessness, the experience of marginalisation, is not, of course, confined to Third World countries. Its manifestations are sometimes more starkly obvious in these societies but relative deprivation impacts on health in Western societies as well: poverty and ill-health go together in all societies (see Chapter Seven).

What to make of 'participation' and the exhortations of agencies and professionals in the context of powerlessness?

We now understand better the processes of marginalisation which is basically the removal of people from decision-making and any significant power and control over their own lives. There have been historical and economic processes of 'departicipation'. For many poor people in the Third World life is a matter of survival on a day-to-day basis; O'Sullivan gives the example of such a situation in Guatemala but the reality is similar in many countries where participation has been promoted: 'Guatemala has a critical problem with the distribution of land: 75 per cent of the farmholdings have an average of 1.3 hectares, while some 100 large farms occupy 15 per cent of all the available agricultural land, with 5000 hectares each' (O'Sullivan, 1980: 82).

What can it mean for a peasant on the edge of survival in a basically unjust and dehumanising situation to be told by a development or health worker to 'participate'? For many people in industrialised Europe, also, jobless and bereft of real choices concerning their lives, it might seem almost obscene to be encouraged by middle-class professionals to 'participate'. In the life context of a family living in a high-rise apartment block and subsisting on social security, the preoccupation must inevitably also be one of survival.

Poverty and powerlessness go together. In the situation of exclusion from participation in the means of production and livelihood (for example from working the land or from jobs), the practice of participation in development or health is difficult to envisage. When participation began to become the key word of development workers and writers in the 1970s, resistance was encountered. The promotion of people's participation in development as a 'basic right and basic human need' sounded somewhat hollow. There was a rejection by some of the use (or 'abuse') of the vocabulary of participation. A good example of this was seen at the World Conference on Agrarian Reform and Rural Development held in Rome in 1979. The documents of this conference were full of the vocabulary of participation:

> Participation by the people in the institutions and systems which govern their lives is a basic human right ... Rural development strategies can realise their full potential only through the motivation, active involvement and organisation at the grass roots level of rural people, with special emphasis on the least advantaged, in conceptualising and designing policies and programmes (Rome Declaration on Agrarian Reform and Rural Development, 1979, in FAO, Ideas and Action, 1980:1).

A counter group set up its conference in Rome at the same time and produced its own declaration, 'On Agrarian Conflict'. It denounced the abuse of the vocabulary of participation saying that it had become a smokescreen for oppressive practices:

> Genuine participation of people in taking hold of development problems is what is being resisted, in many cases outlawed, in the very countries claiming to be for 'participation'. The language of participation is then being used by governments to draw attention away from their suppression of their people's right to organise. (Statement on poster issued by Rome Declaration on Agrarian Conflict, 1979).

The use of a vocabulary of participation, as well as a look at the history of programmes claiming to be participatory, must lead to the examination of decision-making structures (and therefore power structures) within a given community or state. If there is a contemporary call for people to participate, does this mean an acknowledgement on the part of those promoting the idea that those they are addressing have not been participating in the past? The main reasons for this non-participation can be seen to be, according to one's point of view, either some innate inability on the majority's part, some internal deficiency preventing them from being able to participate, or the structures – economic and social – which hinder this participation. Then the question is raised, as it must be: are people allowed to participate in any active sense? In any decision-making? Have they, in the past, been given the power to participate? Are they being given this power now? The promotion of people's participation focuses our attention on power and how it is shared; how power is shared between people in the community and how it is shared between professionals and their clients in the community. As one commentator says, 'participation means sharing, not only of duties, but also of power and privileges'. She goes on to say that the logical consequence of promoting power-sharing is that those who have power must learn to renounce some of it: 'since power and privilege have hardly ever been renounced voluntarily, the concept of a truly participatory society may necessitate in the final analysis the struggle for power' (Traitler, 1974:4). From this perspective, participation is clearly about power-sharing. Here we have an example of the usefulness of Cohen and Uphoff's taxonomy: existing balances of power are not unduly disturbed by poor people participating in the implementation or benefits of projects or programmes, but the promotion of participation as decision-making and evaluation begins to raise the question of control over resources and the direction of programmes and, inevitably, this raises the possibility of conflict of some kind.

The research group, the United Nations Research Institute for Social Development (UNRISD) was quite clear about the power dimension of people's participation and defined participation as the organised effort to increase control over resources and regulative institutions on the part of groups and movements of those hitherto excluded from such control (UNRISD, 1979: 8). Such an understanding has no difficulty in incorporating a notion of conflict (understood, of course, in the sense of the confrontation and optimistically, perhaps, the resolution of different positions without any necessary use of force). Mathias Stiefel, one of the directors of this programme says that a definition of participation such as this, which acknowledges a potentially conflictual process, a redistribution of power, 'calls for a scientific analysis which gives due recognition to political factors, social forces and the role of class in historical processes of social change' (UNRISD, 1981: 3).

He goes on to say that the acknowledgement that participation is about power involves a 'mainly conflictual, sometimes possibly violent, "encounter-model" that questions established relations of power among social groups' (*idem*). He sees this as being a difficult definition for a UN body such as his own to adopt. In the area of health care and the promotion of people's participation it could be argued that it is a difficult definition for the medical establishment to adopt.

UNRISD makes the useful distinction between 'systems-maintaining' and 'systems-transforming' participation (UNRISD, 1979: 20). Systems-maintaining participation is the kind aimed at making people more 'responsive' to development policies of authorities. In such a mode of participation there would be little genuine decision-making on the part of communities. Systems-transforming participation would be the promotion of people's involvement in a way which would allow a concern with structural change and a genuine democratic transfer of power to 'those hitherto excluded' from control of any significant kind (those groups which are sometimes described as 'marginalised'). In such systems-transforming participation there is an effort to allow some significant decision-making to 'participants'. The promotion of participation from this latter point of view calls for an examination of the obstacles to it, not first of all in the so-called 'backward' attitudes of those called to participate; rather, in the first instance, obstacles must be acknowledged in the groups which stand to profit from the distribution of power and resources in the present system. Only this kind of participation can claim to be genuine. By implication, systems-maintaining participation should be seen rather as manipulation and incorporation (Kidd and Kumar, 1979: 3). It is not difficult, from such a perspective, to see obstacles to participation in the class, race and gender dimensions of organisation of society and so these areas become necessary foci of research on participation. Once again one is struck by the impossibility of separating the three pillars of PHC: an examination of participation leads inevitably to considerations of equity and, of course, the lack of equity in all social arrangements, including those concerning health. The promotion of participation is at the same time a promotion of a process of equity. There is much here, in the understanding and promotion of participation in the world of development thinking and practice, for health workers to reflect upon.

Participation by the community was promoted in community development and *animation rurale* programmes of the 1950s and

1960s. Again, there are lessons to be drawn by health workers from this experience. These programmes were devised by the colonising powers, Britain and France, to promote development in the soon-to-be independent countries of Africa and Asia. Then, as now, there were great expectations of community participation – the vocabulary might have been slightly different, but the ideas were the same: the community was to become more actively involved in the development process, become more the motor-force and less the passive receiver. As Holdcroft, one of the original promoters of the process in the world of Anglo-Saxon influence, puts it, community development (CD) should be seen as a process, a movement which, among other things, 'involves people on a community basis in the solution of their common problems' (Holdcroft, 1978: 10) but he goes on to say that, though participation was a major goal of the strategy of CD, it 'proved a most difficult and elusive goal to attain ... The CD experience indicates that, if the rural poor are to be helped, the structural barriers to greater equity must be addressed and this because the local elite almost invariably managed to profit disproportionately from development programmes' (ibid, 30). There are certainly lessons here for the promoters of Primary Health Care and health for all: equity and participation must go hand in hand and if you promote strategies of participation you must be ready to counter-act the tendency whereby the benefits get highjacked by those already with power and advantage.

Moreover, it is quite clear from the comments of such commentators that the vocabulary of 'participation' or 'self-reliance' was used by many of the promoters of community development in colonial times as a means of masking central government's abdication of responsibility for some of the needs of the rural population. The rhetoric was progressive but it was sometimes a smokescreen for relative neglect. Without a genuine commitment to equity, to redressing existing imbalances in society, talk of participation can be rather suspect. Likewise, in Francophone Africa there was, in the experience of the promotion of 'participation' in *animation rurale* programmes, despite the vocabulary, no real sharing of power. The exception was, perhaps, in Senegal (Moulton, 1979), where initially a strong leadership saw *animation rurale* as a genuinely socialist movement, building some power-sharing structures at the grassroots which allowed for people's participation. Popular involvement was to be encouraged in the whole range of development activities, including health. The result? No one can say that these original policies of participation failed in Senegal. For several years people were educated for participation, villages were organised with a sort of grassroots democracy, with channels of communication with government and services. There can be no doubt that some genuine 'bottom-up' development took place: 'planned development for and by the masses' (Cisse, 1964: 47). The programmes, however, were stopped, the leadership was jailed and Leopold Senghor assumed total control of the country, dismantling the structures of participation and power-sharing at the community level. Ultimately, *animation rurale* was replaced by *promotion humaine*, a programme which views development as a technical matter to be transferred to the peasant masses rather than, as in the original notion of *animation*, involving people in participatory processes of decision-making (Moulton, 1979: 172). The participatory vocabulary of *animation rurale* remains to this day in several francophone African countries (as well as *animation urbaine* and *animation feminine*) but the structures which allowed for some taking of power at the grassroots have long since been dismantled. Systems-transforming participation has been replaced by a systems-maintaining version. The promotion of participation ran into difficulties when those 'hitherto excluded from power' began to exercise some democratic rights and take decisions. The obstacles to the process lay mainly in the resistance of those who would have to let go of some power.

A most useful summing-up of the promotion of people's participation or involvement in social processes has been given by Sherry R. Arnstein. What she wrote in the early 1970s in the context of citizen participation in the United States should be compulsory reading for those health workers who use the vocabulary of people's participation or community involvement in health in any context:

> Participation ... is a revered idea that is virtually applauded by everyone. The applause is reduced to polite handclaps, however, when this principle is advocated by the have-nots ... And when the have-nots define participation as a redistribution of power, the American consensus of the fundamental principle explodes into many shades of outright racial, ethnic, ideological and political opposition (Arnstein, 1971: 71).

Arnstein illustrated the nature of participation by drawing up a 'ladder of citizen participation'. Like the taxonomy of Cohen and Uphoff, this provides a very useful gauge of what kind of participation is being talked about in any given situation. She describes eight rungs on the ladder of participation. At the bottom are manipulation and therapy forms of participation, really non-participation. Then there are informing, consultation and placation forms of participation, better called degrees of tokenism. Finally, there are partnership, delegated power and citizen control, all of which she sees as being genuine forms of citizen power and worthy of the name participation (ibid, 70). As health workers take up the vocabulary of 'community involvement in health', they could do well to ask themselves which of these kinds of participation they are interested in promoting, beyond the rhetoric.

We have less excuse now for being naïve in the matter of participation. We know it is about power and decision-making on matters which people deem to be significant for them as well as the structures which facilitate this process. Previous promotion of people's involvement, like community development and *animation rurale*, have demonstrated that participation involves some form of conflict, not necessarily violent, but nevertheless some readiness to take on board adjustments called for in redistribution of power. This was often unacceptable to those who already had power and benefited from the status quo and so the vocabulary remained but only as a smokescreen for non-participatory programmes.

The experience of participation in the field of development has shown that, for it to be meaningful, some structures are necessary, some forum for people to be able to get together to voice common concerns and aims. Participation cannot only be about individual involvement; especially for marginalised and relatively powerless people, strength has always been in numbers, in the collective. For participation to occur, there must be a channel for it, some mechanism for people to gather together to share their ideas and to plan some action (Traitler, 1974, Korten, 1980, Martin, 1983). Traitler says that the two essential steps in the participation process are, firstly, gathering together and talking and, secondly, organising for power in such groups. This grouping, she says, is necessary, 'to help people to organise means to create an opportunity for people to participate in development by building some kind of equal position and by providing a framework in which to participate' (Traitler, 1974: 12–13). It is interesting that some versions of people's participation which are promoted in the West, such as the promotion of people's charters, for health or otherwise, carefully exclude the collective dimension of participation and reduce it to some humanisation of the bureaucratic links between the individual and the system. The African proverb comes to mind: one straw alone is not strong, but many straws together are unbreakable.

Some recent health-policy documents give the impression of having discovered participation and express the same enthusiasm for it that was expressed by promoters of community development and *animation rurale* programmes several decades ago. It would seem reasonable, however, to anticipate considerable difficulty in the promotion of community involvement in health and a certain amount of opposition if what we are talking about is any real sharing of power. Power-sharing means being able to question the allocation of resources, often by definition a threat to the status quo. Moreover, participation and the medical model do not easily combine; again there is a question of power-sharing, the very basic question of the control over the processes involved in health care. Who holds the power of decision-making in health matters? Political economists will tell us that it is politicians and their masters. This must be true, at least to some extent. But even within the world of health care when there is some scope for 'power-sharing' we must anticipate opposition from health professionals themselves. Participation or even participatory approaches do not feature largely in medical curricula.

Participation and the medical model

The attempt to promote people's participation in health (or, more accurately, in health services) obviously takes on a different complexion according to the country and culture of each place and the nature of their health services. A variety of difficulties will be encountered. But some of the experiences will be similar and shared ones, given the global influence of what we have called the medical model. All serious attempts to promote participation, community involvement in health, especially, in Cohen and Uphoff's terms, significant participation, ie in decision-making and evaluation, will, at one point or another, as we have seen with the promotion of participation in development, come face to face with the inescapable axiom: participation is about power. Participation is about the redistribution of power. This is rarely going to be a totally smooth process, not anywhere, and not in health-care systems either.

In Chapter Two we have seen that Western allopathic medicine has developed according to a model which sees the health professional, most often the doctor, as the powerful and active partner in the professional–client/community relationship. The notion of people's participation in health runs counter to basic medical training. As a WHO study group on community involvement in health services put it,

> To date there is not much evidence that the education of health personnel has changed in ways that will allow them to understand and be committed to CIH as part of their professional activities. This is perhaps because CIH touches on the very relationship between health personnel and their clients and challenges health personnel to question the nature of that relationship (ie to move away from the idea of provider/recipient to one of partnership (WHO, 1991: 20).

Wherever those entrusted with promoting participation have been formed in systems moulded by the Western medical engineering model they will inevitably run into the contradiction that they themselves have been trained in a way of thinking and acting which is non-participatory. As has already been said, promoting patient and community participation is not a subject that features in many medical curricula. As Briggs and Banahan point out, medical training at present tends to put the doctor in an authoritarian relationship with the patient (and, by extension, with the community). The way both client and practitioner see their encounter has been conditioned in such a way that the patient is ascribed and often readily assumes a passive role. The place for participation in decision-making is not very large in this perspective: 'This intensive focus on pathophysiology de-emphasises the patient ... The physician's position as the one who is in complete charge has been implicated in the decrease of the patient's participation in their own health care' (Briggs and Banahan, 1990: 395). These authors suggest that there is need for a more 'reciprocal or mutually participative relationship' between doctor and patient and, by extension, one could say with the community. The active pursuit of the participation dimension of PHC would make such a reciprocity essential.

Of course, there are health professionals whose work involves encouraging participation, and who spend considerable energy on the difficult task of encouraging individuals and communities to assume a more active role in deciding what their priority health needs are and selecting strategies for meeting these needs. But most participation by individuals and the community in their dealings with the health profession is in implementation – carrying out actions – and also in benefits. Participation in decision-making and evaluation is much more difficult for the medical profession to promote.

The professional mentality promoted by the practice of diagnosing and prescribing does not seem to allow much scope for the client to participate in decision-making and evaluation. But this is only true if we act upon a very limited view of ill-health and medical services and indeed, of the health professional–patient encounter. If there *were* a pill for every ill, as the caricature of the medical model suggests, then of course there is not much room for people's participation in the healing process except explaining (giving their individual or collective case history to the doctor) and then complying faithfully with the treatment once this has been determined by the doctor. Of course, there is no pill for every ill. Sometimes a clear and accurate diagnosis is called for, as, for example if someone is suffering from tuberculosis or a heart condition. If the patient is fortunate, she/he will meet a doctor who is a good medical scientist with the skills to correctly diagnose and treat the problem. But in many states of ill-health it is not possible to have a clear, simple diagnosis. The doctrine of specific aetiology suggests looking for the main cause, preferably a pathogen that can be identified and eliminated. But often this does not reflect the complex reality of disease. Moreover, even if a major 'cause' can be identified, sometimes no simple 'cure' can be forthcoming. For example, many minor conditions of ill-health in Western societies are ascribed to viral complaints. Since antibiotics have no efficacy in the treatment of viruses, the doctor is often at a loss to know what to 'prescribe'; there *is* no pill. Furthermore, if the complaint is not just simply physical, but the condition is embedded in a web of physical, economic and social circumstances which at the very least predispose the patient to physical illness, the medical practitioner is again often at a loss. Good doctors will rebel at the suggestion that the medical model leads to unnecessary prescription of drugs like antibiotics and many spend considerable time in trying to deal more holistically with their clients. But the research evidence is there to show that the medical model can lead to the prescribing of a 'remedy', even when it is unnecessary and sometimes positively unhelpful. It is difficult to believe that what has been shown concerning the over-prescribing of antibiotics in Britain in the 1980s is very different from the situation in other countries: 'doctors continue to prescribe thousands of drugs that are inappropriate, unnecessary, dangerous or ineffective. So, for example, according to a Symposium held at the Royal Society of Medicine in 1983 a massive fifty per cent of the prescriptions written for antibiotics were thought to be quite unnecessary or totally inappropriate' (Coleman, 1988: 47).

The cause for this unhelpful situation cannot be laid totally at the door of individual doctors or indeed the health profession. It is wrong for society to medicalise all problems of ill-health and expect doctors to 'cure' everything. But there is a strong tradition within medicine which we have described earlier, which tends to perpetuate just such a medicalisation of the causes of, and so the remedies for, ill-health. It seems fair enough to say, then, that the engineering model or paradigm within which doctors are led to conceptualise their work does not readily see a place for people's active participation in the way we have described. The model actually encourages a distance from the patient. Maguire says that by stressing physical interventions to remedy underlying disease processes, the bio-engineering approach in medical care 'usually ignores patients' emotional responses to illness and encourages doctors to maintain a distance from their patients' (Maguire, 1984: 162). Participation is about the sharing of power, as we have seen, and in the medical encounter, all the power is with the doctor. Maguire suggests that the reason for the encouragement of the distance he talks of is to strengthen the doctors' image as authority figures and with the purpose of increasing their power to reassure patients.

It has been suggested that the existing medical model has an in-built 'problem-orientation'. By this is meant that it is focused almost exclusively on the identification and correction of health-related problems. Although this has contributed much to the understanding and management of acute and curable illnesses, these 'represent a smaller and smaller proportion of current medical practice' in Western society. What they propose is a 'goal-oriented' approach to medical care which 'is more applicable to the care of patients with chronic incurable illnesses, that more comfortably includes the principles of health promotion and disease prevention, that is better suited to interdisciplinary teamwork, and that allows for increased involvement of patients in their own health care' (Mold et al, 1991: 46–47). In other words, even within Western society, the limitations of the perspectives and approach of scientific medicine too narrowly conceived are being felt by practitioners who are declaring the need for another model which would allow, *inter alia*, greater space for patients' participation in the task of dealing with health matters.

Primary Health Care and community involvement in health

As we have said, one of the reasons for a move towards a broader understanding of health and health care was the frustration felt by many practitioners of conventional Western medicine; their experience of the limitations of the reactive mode of operation and a narrow biological perspective of health services. The PHC approach acknowledges and is itself part of the incorporation in health-care planning of a wider view of the problems of ill-health – wider circles of investigation, the move from microscope to macroscope – and the need to bring the patient and the public into more of a decision-making role. Doctors and other health workers on their own may not be able to 'cure' problems in the social and economic spheres, but to acknowledge this limitation is perhaps the first step towards a more effective healing process and certainly helps towards a participatory mode of working. It is important to repeat that many doctors and other health workers who have experience of working with patients in the areas of community health as well as disciplines such as mental health and orthopaedics have had to learn to listen and often to work in partnership with their clients. They have learned a participatory mode of work.

Primary Health Care says communities have a right and duty to participate in decision-making concerning their health and the services provided: 'The people have the right and duty to participate individually and collectively in the planning and implementation of their health care' (Alma Ata Declaration, IV). The thread of participation is a major one in Alma Ata's proposals for health policy; it is an emphasis which it is impossible to escape. There can be no doubt that what PHC envisages as participation or community involvement in health cannot be equated with participation only in implementation of projects or simply in benefits of programmes, but is much more what Cohen and Uphoff call significant participation, that is, in decision-making and evaluation: 'PHC requires and promotes maximum community and individual self-reliance and participation in the planning, organisation, operation and control of primary health care, making fullest use of local, national and other available resources; and to this end develops through appropriate education the ability of communities to participate' (Alma Ata Declaration, VII, 5).

Here we have a major challenge to the health systems as they come into contact with the community; the essence of the call is to be much more proactive than simply reactive and to be proactive in a way which does not consist in simply and authoritatively telling the individual or community what is wrong with their health and what must be done to improve it. Promoting active decision-making by the community may well be a difficult task for public health specialists whose main tool is classical epidemiology, given what we have already said about the professional practice and training of such specialists which tends to encourage a certain distance from people's demands, from asking people what they feel and want, from people's active participation. Primary Health Care is supposed to address the main health problems in the community in a way which promotes maximum participation. This must mean that the perceptions, aspirations and needs (self-perceived) of communities are to be a major concern in health planning. If we acknowledge people's right to participate in evaluation and planning, then it should be possible and even necessary to talk of a 'participatory epidemiology'. But the fact is that we rarely hear such expressions. They do not fit with what we have come to understand to be the scope and method of the work of epidemiologists. According to their training, they are ready to analyse data on morbidity and mortality and to suggest correlations and trends. But they have much less preparation in the skills of asking the community what their perceptions of their needs are, what they think of the services provided, nor the skills necessary to enable the community to be involved in future planning. Western scientific medicine sees the community as the aggregation of the (sick or potentially sick) individuals in it. It equips its practitioners to diagnose and tell, not to listen and plan in partnership. Participation means the sharing of power and this is something most doctors are not trained to do even if they are willing. When we talk in Chapter Nine of the new kind of professional demanded by the PHC approach this is a point to which we will have to return.

Part of Cohen and Uphoff's research into programmes promoting people's participation included an examination of some health programmes and they conclude: 'The basic structure and philosophy of health care has been built on a narrow system of technical specialisation and professionalism that puts patients in a subordinate and dependent status and does not require that persons take responsibility for their own health' (Cohen and Uphoff, 1979: 237). In their examination of health projects claiming to be 'participatory' the same researchers say that their findings show that often the same technico-medical mode of operation applies when the health professional turns his or her attention to the community rather than the individual. What is looked for is a sort of collective 'patient compliance' with medical interventions in the community. The chance for participation in health seems slight.

Participation, or community involvement in health, is one of the three major demands of PHC as we have already seen. People have not only a *duty* to participate in matters concerning their health care, but a positive *right* to do so (Alma Ata). Unfortunately, it comes as no surprise that participation in such programmes which claim to be PHC has often followed the same pattern as participation in development movements such as community development and *animation rurale*, in other words, the way of rhetoric and dilution. Moreover, it would be naive to imagine that the mere adoption of a vocabulary of participation is going to remove the obstacles to that participation which are inherent in the medical model. To ask people trained in the skills of medical diagnosis and treatment – top-down medicine – to suddenly become the agents of people's involvement in significant decisions about their own health is expecting rather a lot. The philosophy of PHC, and therefore of people's participation in health, is implemented by people trained in non-participatory ways of thinking and doing. It is no wonder that beyond the vocabulary there has often been little action. This has often led to cynicism about the idea and even outright rejection. The history of the promotion of participation in Community Development has shown us that we should indeed be cautious, not only in promoting participation, but in presuming that the major obstacles in the way of it 'working' always lie in the alleged backwardness of people in the community. Some of the major obstacles to people's participation in health are to be found in the attitudes and practice of the medical profession.

In an evaluation of 52 USAID-sponsored programmes of PHC, all proclaiming to promote people's participation, an assessment of this participation found that there was a considerable amount of community involvement in 'activities directly related to service delivery' – presumably the kind of participation which Cohen and Uphoff would call participation in implementation. The evaluation found little evidence of what these researchers would call significant participation, the kind which involves communities in decision-making and evaluation: 'Communities rarely have a role in defining major features of programmes, or even in determining what their own activities and responsibilities will be. Most communities are presented with a defined package of responsibilities and a predetermined format for executing those tasks' (Parlato and Favin, 1982: 37). An understanding of the medical model and the conditioning it involves in the mentalities of both health worker and communities can help us understand why participation in health programmes, even those proclaiming themselves to be PHC programmes, gets presented as a 'package' to be delivered to the community/patient by the health professional; the community 'participates' by complying. The literature yields little in the way of successful participation in PHC programmes. This is despite the predictable vocabulary, as for example in the Riga document from WHO, looking at ten years of PHC: 'PHC cannot achieve coverage and effectiveness without the full involvement of communities' (WHO, 1988).

Wisner's look at PHC programmes leads him to depressing conclusions and to wonder 'Why language so explicitly non-technical, comprehensive and participatory is implemented as its opposite'. He goes on to say that 'one obviously not very helpful answer is that inertia in health-care systems is as great or even greater than it is in other institutions' (Wisner, 1988: 58). This is to underestimate and perhaps even misunderstand the inbuilt resistance of the medical model to participation. It is not simply what Wisner describes as inertia which confronts the demand of participation in health systems, what we are dealing with is a positively anti-participatory mode of thinking and action inculcated by the medical engineering model. Unless this is understood there is little hope for participation in PHC. This is in no way to deny the fundamental argument of Wisner and others that PHC often gets interpreted in a weak, non-participatory manner because strong versions of PHC call for a readiness for structural change, the sharing of political power and this is an undertaking which will meet with considerable political opposition. But the critics of weak versions of PHC should acknowledge the great strength of medical opposition to participation which mirrors and in a sense is part of the social and political opposition to a strong PHC with its emphasis on real participation and a move towards equity. The two sources of opposition, political and medical establishment can often work in tandem. Advocates of alternative health care systems must see that this means that there is a double opposition to people's involvement in health care, in decision-making and evaluation. This is as true in Europe as it is in so-called developing countries.

Structures for people's participation

For participation to occur, there must be a channel for it, some structures offering a mechanism for people to gather together to share their ideas and to plan some action (Traitler, 1974, Korten, 1980, Martin, 1983). This has led, in health care, to the formation of village and neighbourhood health committees, as well as, in the West, to such structures as the British Community Health Councils and, on a more grassroots level, neighbourhood tenants committees and the like, as well as those groups which we have already described as belonging to the Community Health Movement. Experience has shown that the participatory dimensions must be welded to the equity dimension, otherwise such committees can begin to represent the interests of the relatively more advantaged people in the community who already have a voice. Moreover, it is legitimate to ask how much attention is paid to such groupings and how much are they really intended as mechanisms of ensuring collective 'patient-compliance'? Why have the Community Health Councils in Britain been removed from any decision-making role on Area Health Boards? There are political answers, of course, but the deafening silence of protest from the medical world (the medical world was not up in arms to ensure community representation) is in itself significant. Some health workers have come to realise that participation in health matters cannot easily be separated from participation in other social and development sectors and that they should therefore be ready to work within whatever participatory structures already exist. The inspirational Jamkhed Project in Maharashta in India encourages participation in health matters through Young Farmers Clubs already in existence since these allowed some form of community debate and action (Arole and Arole, 1975). Sometimes PHC programmes have to create such structures, like village or neighbourhood health committees, or to resurrect moribund structures (Macdonald, 1981). In some countries of South America the churches offer what is sometimes the only structure in society which offers people the opportunity to organise around issues such as health, to 'participate' in health matters.

In Indonesia it is reported that structures for popular participation exist at the village level as part of the national PHC programme:

> At the village level, community health development is an integral part of overall village development under the

umbrella of the Village Community Resilience Institute, which is the forum of all development activities requiring intersectoral collaboration ... Community participation is achieved by encouraging local people to become involved in analysing problems, formulating plans of operation, deciding priorities, implementing healthy lifestyles, and participating in manpower development, fundraising, and the supply of equipment (Yahya and Roesin, 1990: 136–7).

One is always cautious about the depth of participation when described in such non-conflictual terms by government officials (as in the above example) but there is no doubt that there have been structures allowing some form of people's participation in health matters in many countries attempting to follow the policies laid down at Alma Ata. In the particular case of Indonesia, Johnston suggests that although equity has not been a major concern in the development strategy in that country in recent years, there is nevertheless a basis for 'developing PHC services through which low-income communities can participate in determining the direction and momentum' (Johnston, 1983: 189). This is an important point, because there is a danger that the promotion of the three pillars of PHC can appear to set standards which are impossibly high. The art of the promotion of PHC is to seek to implement PHC policies within whatever room for manoeuvre is available.

There are many lessons for Western societies to learn from the PHC approach as it is being practised in countries of the Third World. Industrialised societies are generally way behind in terms of the acknowledgement of people's right to participate and the fostering of structures of community involvement in health and the development of people's health organisations. It is clear that industrialised societies in the West do not have a culture which readily allows for group participation; the nuclear family often lives its life in isolation from its neighbours. Structures which would allow for the promotion of participation are not always immediately obvious. But if the medical – or health – profession was working in a participatory manner in its contact with individuals, there would be a predisposition to encourage group and community involvement in health. This is part of the challenge, the acknowledgement that health care is not only the business of the health profession, it is also people's business, a partnership with people. But there is more to this challenge posed by the PHC approach: there are other pillars of the PHC approach. One of these is the acknowledgement that other sectors contribute, sometimes largely to people's health. The PHC approach says that this contribution has to be recognised and incorporated into health planning and policies; intersectoral collaboration is the subject of the next chapter.

Chapter Six

The Second Pillar:
Intersectoral Collaboration

One of the three pillars of the Primary Health Care approach is the policy directive that the health sector should work together with other sectors which contribute to health. This is what is meant by the policy of intersectoral collaboration. A necessary precondition for any movement in this direction is the acknowledgement by those working in health that other sectors have an important role to play in the establishment of good health both of individuals and of the community at large. The consequences of this acknowledgement must be not only respect for the contribution of other sectors but also the readiness to collaborate with them in the management and planning of health services.

An intersectoral approach to health-care activities is a logical consequence of a broad understanding of the multiple factors which contribute to health and disease: just as there are many factors in the personal and social environment of individuals and communities which impact on their health and disease and are more directly in the sphere of influence of other sectors, so health workers should be ready to collaborate with the professionals in these other sectors. Health workers do not have a monopoly of health work. In this sense intersectoral collaboration flows directly from the preoccupation with building health rather than medical services.

So much for common sense; unfortunately, there are considerable obstacles in the way of logic and common sense being translated into the daily practice of any government sector, including health. All organisations tend to develop their own bureaucratic mode of operation and we have long accepted the workings of bureaucracy as necessary means of living together in society. But bureaucracies tend to have a non-integrated and even a fragmented or piecemeal approach to development and social organisation. They need mechanisms of decision-making and organisation which often involve committees and hierarchical procedures and these institutions lead easily to formalism, a process in which these procedures and even the organisations can become ends in themselves, at the worst self- perpetuating and all with their own laws and sub-culture. In Third World countries, ministries of agriculture and education, to say nothing of ministries of health, have their own bureaucratic procedures which do not readily dispose those working in them to work with other sectors. Social work departments and health departments in Western societies sometimes find themselves working with the same persons and certainly the same communities as clients but are prevented from working together on account of differing bureaucratic procedures. At the level of the communities which such bureaucracies are intended to serve such non-collaboration can mean individuals and groups having contact with various authorities sometimes with conflicting and therefore confusing messages.

Most of the countries of the Third World have inherited and developed bureaucratic organisation from the West and there are many accounts of the cumbersome nature of bureaucratic procedures. But there are exemplary rays of light in the bureaucratic gloom of some countries from which the West could usefully learn if it had the mind. In Bangladesh, some two decades ago, Akhtar Hameed Khan developed the Comilla Programme which was based on the notion that different government agencies or bureaucracies could learn to work in partnership with communities if they themselves were trained to work in a more integrated manner. Integrated development was what Khan promoted, with considerable success, at least in Comilla. Much more attention should be given by national governments as well as the international development agencies to his work and the re-organisation of the bureaucratic structures of government which it involved, to make these more responsive to people's needs and more organs of development than brakes upon it. Of course, in Bangladesh as elsewhere, the disintegrating force of bureaucracies was and still is at work and the efforts to promote the relative success of the Comilla programme to the whole country ran into considerable difficulty (Khan, 1985).

It is not only different sectors which have in-built tendencies not to cooperate with one another. Even within the same sector and programme, different divisions can develop working practices in isolation from other sub-sections in their own discipline. In health care this non-integration is a common phenomenon: not only are 'public' health and curative care well separated from each other, it also happens that programmes such as health education can be quite separate from others like immunisation, and mother and child health. What is worse, in the name of PHC, programmes like the control of diarrhoeal diseases are often organised quite separately from sanitation and acute respiratory infections programmes. The discussion of selective versus comprehensive PHC which was the focus of Chapter Four is relevant here: whatever arguments are put forward for or against selecting diseases for technical-medical intervention programmes, there will always be biases towards this segregation coming both from the medical model and from the inherent tendency of bureaucracies to organise separately. One of the ironies in the health world is that the very organisation which has promoted a comprehensive, integrated and intersectoral approach to health care, WHO, has itself been involved in the promotion of programmes which are often selective in practice and separated from one another, all in the name of PHC. Programmes, such as those for diarrhoeal disease control and programmes of acute respiratory infections, to name but two, both emanating from WHO in the name of PHC, tend to develop separate structures, separate hierarchies.

The most unfortunate non-collaboration in the field of health care might well be between clinical and public health. If we see treatment and prevention as the two 'arms' of Western health care systems, we can say that not only has the prevention arm seemed to develop signs of withering in the last half-century, but often neither arm seems to be aware of what the other is doing. The Alma Ata (comprehensive) approach to PHC challenges the health sector to work with other sectors; it also challenges sub-sections within the health sector to work in a more integrated, intra-sectoral manner.

Intersectoral collaboration can be seen as a simple imperative of common sense. The contribution of other sectors of health can hardly be in dispute. Education, housing, water and sanitation, social work, community development and agriculture, to name but a few, have a considerable impact on health. Alma Ata was clear about this: 'PHC involves, in addition to the health sector, all related sectors and aspects of national and community development, in particular agriculture, animal husbandry, food, industry, education, housing, public works, communications and other sectors; and demands the coordinated efforts of all those sectors'

(Alma Ata Declaration, VII, 4). This is strong language from an international body: the Conference not only exhorts, but demands coordination between the sectors.

Education clearly has an important contribution to make to the health status of populations. Some would say that the most significant single intervention one can make in a community in order to improve its health status is to organise educational activities for the women in that community. The real primary health care workers in the world's families are mothers; education of mothers has enormous impact on the health of families. Education supplies not only information, but confidence: 'Education improves a woman's skills for survival and her capacity for self-care and maintenance of good health during pregnancy; it enables her to acquire greater knowledge and learn better child care practices. This behaviour is related more to the confidence she has acquired ... than to what she was actually taught in school (WHO, 1986a: 78).

Sometimes promoters of PHC think that their commitment to education is accounted for by the PHC programme having an educational component (see Chapter Eight). But the imperative of intersectoral collaboration must mean much more for health workers than this. There is considerable evidence of the links between education (especially maternal education) and improved health status: knowledge of this must move the health worker to active collaboration with the education sector.

A longitudinal study in Kenya examining childhood mortality highlighted the importance of such factors as the educational and marital status of the child's mother. Children of mothers of the highest educational level had 65 to 115 per cent lower death risk than children of mothers of the lowest educational level (Kune, 1980). There is some difficulty in separating out the impact on children's health status of different variables like parental income and educational levels and, in any case, these often go together. In many countries, including western countries, educational status is often linked to socio-economic status with both of these impacting on health. A study of the infant mortality rates in the years 1964–66 in the United States found that the rates were in inverse relationship to family income and level of educational achievement of both father and mother: infant mortality was 77 per cent higher for children of mothers who had only elementary school education than for children of mothers who had graduated from college (Kitagawa et al, 1973).

An intersectoral approach obliges the health worker to see the education sector as an important ally in the furthering of the health of individuals and communities. At this level it is not important to decide whether increased levels of education are possible without or more important than increased levels of income; the health worker should be interested in the promotion of both.

One interesting example of intersectoral collaboration between the health and education sectors is the Child-to-Child programme. The basic idea is simple: children are not only potential recipients of health education, they need to be recognised as having themselves an active role in health education and health promotion (Aarons et al, 1970). Children in many societies already have easily recognisable roles in promoting health in their communities; the Child-to-Child programme sets out to build on this fact and to encourage children to be health promoters for their siblings, peers, families and communities.

The role of the quantity and quality of water available to families for cooking and hygiene and the importance of adequate waste disposal are well documented in the promotion of health both in Western society (McKeown, 1976) as well as in so-called developing countries:

> Nearly half of the population of developing countries suffers from health problems related to unsafe water and inadequate sanitation. A survey in 1980 revealed that only 33 per cent of the rural population had safe drinking water compared to 74 per cent of the urban population ... The health consequences of inadequate water supply and sanitation can be drastic. Infant and childhood diarrhoeas alone are estimated to cause 4.5–5 million deaths per year out of some 600–700 million episodes ... improvements in water and sanitation could result in a 25 per cent reduction in morbidity (WHO, 1986a: 101–102).

Such knowledge and information is commonplace in most countries of the Third World and should logically lead to the endorsement of policies of collaboration between health workers and those sectors involved in water and sanitation. Unfortunately, this is not always the case. Walsh and Warren, in their endorsement of the selective approach to PHC rule out the inclusion of water and sanitation programmes in their targeted interventions (Walsh and Warren, 1979). Other commentators find the exclusion of Water and Sanitation programmes very short-sighted in terms of the potential impact for reducing diseases; moreover, 'Studies have shown that rural water supplies are not only reasonably priced, but that they enhance the effectiveness of other development initiatives' (Yacoob et al, 1989: 332).

The importance of adequate and proper food in the promotion of health has already been mentioned in this work; health workers faced with malnutrition find themselves, at least in rural and peri-urban situations, inevitably in the domain of agriculture. Lipton and De Kadt begin their book on agriculture-health linkages by drawing attention to two synergisms affecting morbidity and mortality, in the first instance in Third World countries and secondly in industrialised countries. They show that agricultural products and processes are linked to the main causes of disease and death and also to the ways of preventing them in both sets of societies. In non-industrialised countries we have the synergism (joint action) of malnutrition and infectious diseases which we have already mentioned and which is a major cause of high morbidity and mortality rates especially among children of poor families. Consequently, 'farming circumstances are the main determinant of health among vulnerable groups in developing countries'. The other synergism at work, this time in industrialised countries, and again a major cause of death in these societies is 'between the use of various agricultural products – some beneficial such as fibres, some dangerous such as tobacco – and other elements of the "lifestyle" such as stress, work conditions and sedentary living' (Lipton and de Kadt, 1988: 5).

This second synergism is a main cause of important diseases of the heart, as well as cancers and stroke. In all societies, when health workers look beyond treatment to prevention they are drawn to the need for intersectoral collaboration, in this case, the need to work with the agriculture sector as well as with the food industry sector. Working with, in this case, might mean on occasion having to denounce the latter industry when it indulges in practices injurious to health. The medical model of health tends to see the individual family as having responsibility in the matter of food and health and again it might call for professional courage for the health worker to accept the need to caution not only the consumer but the producer. This expanded role of what we can call health education is indeed part of what is understood as health promotion and this is a topic we will turn to more fully in the chapter on health education (Chapter Eight).

As we have said several times, in impoverished societies and poor sections of all communities diseases are often united in their source: poverty. Malnutrition is linked to infection and infection to malnutrition. Poor housing, poor diet, the lack of choice that comes from lack of money, poor water supply, all these things are linked in a vicious syndrome that promotes ill-health. We have already quoted Ian Kennedy as saying, 'Very many of the people to whom we are readily prepared to ascribe the status "ill" find themselves ill because they are poor, grow up in bad housing, eat poor food, work, if at all, at depressing jobs, and generally exist on the margin of survival' (Kennedy, 1981: 28). Chambers (1983) speaks of 'integrated poverty' and it is clear in the light of what we have been saying of various synergisms that we can also speak of integrated ill-health and disease. The argument that many of the causes of health and ill-health are interlinked is the rationale for intersectoral collaboration, the integration of those services which contribute to health. Once the synergistic relationship between these causes is grasped, their 'working-together', the consequences for policy and planning are obvious: the different sectors which contribute to health need also to work together.

Unfortunately, the needs of the community have not been seen or dealt with in an integrated, intersectoral way. Each service organisation or bureaucracy – and this includes the health service – interprets the needs of people according to the way it sees the world and generally in isolation from other sectors. Sometimes responses to community needs are organised according to the needs of the service sector in question rather than according to the needs of the community. Community needs, in any case, are generally taken to be what the profession understands the community to need rather than those stated by the community as what they perceive as necessary or important. Community assessment often reveals the links between different aspects of life at the grassroot level: people's medical needs, housing needs, water and sanitation and nutritional needs are all interlinked in the life of that one person or community, the recipient of services. It is only on the level of providing of services, the bureaucratic level, that housing, disposal of waste, medical needs etc get divided.

The call or 'demand' for intersectoral collaboration on the part of health workers is extremely logical. Health planners and indeed many other workers from sectors other than health are able to see the theoretical importance and indeed necessity of such collaboration. But once professionals in the health sector take on board the call for such integration and look for ways that they might implement it, they are accepting to be profoundly challenged in their own established way of thinking and acting.

Intersectoral collaboration and the medical model

The famous definition of health by WHO: not just the absence of disease, but the total well-being of individuals and communities, does not diminish the important role of curative care; rather it situates medical care within health care. The focus by the medical profession on disease rather than health, which was dealt with in Chapter Three, brings about an understanding of the work of health services which encompasses the 'inner circles' of causality and remedy to the virtual exclusion of the 'outer circles': the chosen instrument, we have said, is the microscope. But there is need also for a macroscope, a systematic look at the wider circles of causality of disease and health. This would lead to an appreciation of the health-promoting role of other sectors. Medical services can and do function in relative isolation from other sectors; a genuine *health* service would see intersectoral collaboration as normal. The status of medicine is such, however, that it will often take considerable political will for a health system to endorse such a vision and even more to make it operative.

Perhaps it is when health professionals are confronted with clear evidence of the adverse effects of poverty on health that the need to work with other sectors becomes inescapable. This may be the reason that expanded understandings of health and of health care and an intersectoral approach have come mainly from the so-called Third World where poverty and its effects are sometimes more glaringly obvious. At the Child in Need Institute (CINI) outside Calcutta, young doctors explained to me the adjustments they had to make when dealing with undernutrition in the villages around the hospital headquarters: almost as soon as they arrived in the villages for the first time they were asked questions about the relative nutritional merits of different vegetables and problems of cultivation and storage. One young doctor explained how angry such questions had made her since they 'made her look foolish'. Despite her high status as a doctor and after all her years of study, she did not know the answer and was not at first able to direct the questioners to people who did have the right answer. She knew about medicine, not vegetables (CINI, 1988). In Chapter Nine we will examine a little more fully the consequences of the application of PHC principles, from the 'demand' for intersectoral collaboration to the training of health professionals, but there can surely be no doubt that the technico-medical orientation of conventional medicine tends to make intersectoral collaboration seem like a quaint option rather than an essential element of any health work.

Improvements in the living conditions of poor people almost always makes a significant impact on their health status. This is true whether or not the health services have been involved (Marshall and Yanz, 1988). The impact of non-health sectors on health status was enormous in Europe in the last century (McKeown, 1976), when the pattern of ill-health was extraordinarily similar to that of so-called developing countries today (Sanders, 1985). There are very articulate voices in Europe today which argue that the links between poverty and ill-health are there to be observed and too-well documented to be denied (Townsend and Davidson, 1982; Wilkinson, 1992). It is unclear whether this research leads health workers to conceive of their work in broader terms and become involved in the promotion of health through anti-poverty measures.

Just as the call to participation is a call to the health profession to share power with those they seek to help, so the call for intersectoral collaboration is a similar call to the profession to find ways of working with sectors which are known to contribute to people's health. Likewise, just as participation, as we have seen, requires structures to make it operational, so too does intersectoral collaboration. Planning for PHC involves, in addition to creative management of the health sector, the management of regular contact both with community structures and other sectors which contribute to health.

As we saw in Chapter Three, Alma Ata declared the necessity of working with other sectors, thereby making this mandatory for those claiming to be PHC promoters: 'PHC involves, in addition to the health sector, all related sectors and aspects of national and community development, in particular, agriculture, animal husbandry, food, industry, education, housing, public works, communications ... and demands the coordinated efforts of all those sectors' (WHO/UNICEF, 1978). Subsequent documents have argued for this approach, such as *Intersectoral Collaboration for Health* (WHO, 1986a). The document begins by reporting a resolution of the 39th World Health Assembly of May, 1986. Among its calls to member states is the following:

> The 39th World Health Assembly calls on member states to ensure that the training of health professionals at all levels encompasses an adequate awareness of the relationships between environment, living conditions, lifestyles and local health problems in order to enable them to establish a meaningful collaboration with

professionals in other health-related sectors (WHO, 1986a: 10).

The necessary notion of *intra-* as well as *inter*-sectoral collaboration has been put forward. That is to say, integrated efforts for health make sense but even within the health sector there is not as much collaboration between the different sub-sectors as there might be. Intra-sectoral collaboration in practice would mean the effort to promote joint planning between mother and child health programmes and Family Planning programmes, between general practitioners and social work departments and so forth.

The matter of selective or comprehensive PHC has already been discussed. Selective versions of PHC, by promoting targeted audiences and individual conditions, risk considerable overlap. The organisation of PHC programmes into separate interventions is a further example of the disintegrating tendency of bureaucracies, sadly applicable also to the organisation of PHC. As we have said, it is not unknown to have Diarrhoeal Disease programmes and Respiratory Infection programmes working in the same areas but not in an integrated manner. Once again we see the simple logic of integration, of collaboration. In a situation of limited resources, is not intersectoral and intrasectoral collaboration an imperative?

Of course, in practice, in the field, logic is not always easy to follow, in this case within the framework of existing bureaucracies. As one practitioner put it: 'We have a few problems (in the implementation of PHC). The first is integration. We have about seven vertical programmes like Tuberculosis Control, Immunisation, Environmental Health etc. ... But these workers have refused to join me as one body to deliver services to the community' (Liberian health worker, 1987). The need to work with other sectors is expressed not only by individuals in the field. One of the notable advocates of PHC in the context of South East Asia, Dr. Amorn Nondusatu, in his keynote address to the 32nd SEAMO-TROPMED Regional Seminar in 1990 has also noted very clearly the necessity of such an approach, following logically from the realisation that 'the health sector alone cannot achieve significant and lasting improvement (in health)' (Mercado, 1990: 340).

If there is a need to talk of intersectoral collaboration or multidimensional and multidisciplinary approaches, it is because until recently these have been rare phenomena. There have been piecemeal and discrete approaches to people's development and health. All service sectors, including health and education can be seen as being involved in communication exercises: they are in contact with individuals, with communities. They all have, explicitly or otherwise, the idea of passing on information or skills or beneficial attitudes. Despite the intention of these sectors, what one witnesses is fragmented and sometimes contradictory messages. Even when dealing with the same subject, for example, what one might think of as the relatively simple subject of nutrition, several sectors can give very conflicting messages. The rational response to contradictory messages is to resist them. One of the major obstacles to successful health communication is often this lack of integration with other sectors. An example is perhaps useful.

Juala was a hard-working mother of five children. She and her family members were peasant farmers. Their village was one of those included in the health extension programme of their district. Twice a month a mobile clinic visited their village to run a MCH (mother and child health) programme for the local mothers. The nurse ran a growth monitoring session, giving the mothers, including Juala, advice about weaning foods and other nutritional matters. Four out of five of Juala's children seemed to be undernourished and therefore prone to infection. Sometimes the nurse became somewhat irritated because Juala seemed to ignore this advice. The health promotion message was not complicated and the nurse was definitely going beyond a narrow medical model: Juala was encouraged to grow a few groundnuts and some green vegetables near her home and to combine these in the daily diet of the younger children. But not only did Juala not seem to listen, after several months she stopped coming to the sessions and contrived to be out of the village when the mobile clinic came. The nurse had many examples of such frustrating behaviour on the part of her clients.

What the nurse did not realise was the Juala's withdrawal, far from being a manifestation of 'backwardness' or hardheadedness, was a completely rational response. Her village was also visited on a regular basis by an agricultural extension team. This team encouraged the women of the village to keep small livestock like chickens and goats near the house. The women of the village realised, from experience, that the message of the MCH clinic about vegetable-growing near the home and the message about goats and chickens were incompatible. The one 'solution' would eat the other. The men in the village were more interested in the possibility of occasional meat. It turned out that at least five departments or sectors were offering mothers advice related to nutrition. No doubt these sectors imagined that their messages were mutually reinforcing but they were experienced as different and sometimes downright contradictory (Macdonald, 1988).

In Europe, one of the best known examples of intersectoral collaboration is that presented by the North Karelia project in Finland (WHO, 1981), a programme of community control of cardiovascular disease. From the outset, the programme was conceived as being a *health* programme which would necessarily involve sectors other than the medical sector. The project has worked with the food industry and influenced it in a very positive way; it has also been involved with schools from the beginning and with voluntary organisations. This has included substituting the marketing of local vegetables and berries for dairy farming, as it was found that the consumption of dairy products was reduced with the new dietary habits encouraged by the programme. There is some difficulty in measuring the impact of programmes with various strategies such as this one in a country where the overall health status is improving anyhow (RUHBC, 1989). But what success there has been (statistics show that mortality from ischaemic heart disease has been reduced by 22 per cent in North Karelia compared with 11 per cent in the rest of Finland) must be due in part to the medical profession's commitment to work with other health-related sectors (Nissinen et al, 1988).

Buttfield et al. tell us that their experience in Australia shows that the diseases most often confronting family doctors or GPs in industrialised countries are chronic conditions such as diabetes and doctors are more able to manage these conditions if they work in conjunction with professionals from other sectors (Buttfield et al, 1990).

In the area of maternal health there is often a tendency to separate maternal health services from other health programmes and of course from other development activities in the community. After studying a variety of situations, Fraser and Meli come to the conclusion that public health workers should focus on intersectoral programmes at the community level. Such programmes can create structures which allow women to organise around health issues. Their conclusion is that the best means of promoting maternal health in Third World countries is to promote sustainable development programmes since these have the greatest potential to produce lasting changes in the risks of childbearing: the sort of PHC they envisage is therefore clearly of the comprehensive type (Fraser et al, 1990).

The link between intersectoral collaboration and participation

Nondasatu shows one of the ways in which the two demands of participation and intersectoral collaboration are linked. If health workers promote people's participation seriously, they will inevitably be in touch with groups of people who are being encouraged to express their needs and then helped to meet these needs in partnership with professionals. If you listen to people express their needs and attempt to help bridge the gap between needs and available help and resources you have to acknowledge the limits of any one profession to meet these needs: intersectoral respect and collaboration are the inevitable outcome. Nondusatu gives the example of his own country, Thailand, where working with communities led health workers to realise that in the struggle for survival, communities often have needs more immediately urgent to them than health needs. These primary felt needs have to be taken into account; people, he says, are mostly interested in livelihood projects. Health was only one of their felt basic needs; but by taking their expressed needs seriously one has a credibility when dealing with their health problems (Mercado, 335). A broad vision of health, an openness to participation and the expression of people's needs leads to a 'multidimensional' approach, the working together of the various service sectors involved. Part of the genius of Akhter Hameed Khan, whose work in Bangladesh has already been mentioned, was to see this need for structures which allowed for both integration and people's participation.

The logical argument in favour of integration, intersectoral collaboration, is clear. Verbal support for the principle is readily given. The literature, however, reveals little in the way of documentation and research into the practice. An interesting study of the intersectoral dimension of a small local PHC programme in Dahu, China, which combined with apparently considerable success such components as health education, environmental sanitation and housing, suggests the importance of both local structures which permit participation as well as political support: 'political commitment is essential in fostering the intersectoral coordination that supports the process of community participation. Such a multisectoral approach is possible only through an enlightened leadership and citizenry that is informed about the benefits of PHC' (Hongelian et al, 1991: 26).

Once again we see that in the area of intersectoral collaboration we are moving away from the idea of selective medical programmes. Comprehensive PHC programmes involve a multi-disciplinary approach almost by definition. There are not only philosophical and moral arguments in favour of working together. There is evidence that the pillars of PHC are mutually reinforcing. A study comparing programmes in Togo and Indonesia, both of which programmes encouraged people's participation in the building of a safe water system, shows a link between the participatory safe water schemes and people's involvement in an immunisation programme. An empirical comparison of villages with and without community-based water projects in the two countries shows that between 25 and 30 per cent more children are immunised in villages with community-based water projects than in comparison villages which have not (Eng et al, 1984).

The study of Yacoob et al., already mentioned, shows the links between people's participation and the intersectoral approach: they give the example of a Nigerian programme in which the community, given the chance to participate, expressed their need for clean safe water (Yacoob et al, 1989). Briscoe (Briscoe, 1984) suggests that if poor women were given the chance to voice their needs, water programmes would be a high priority for them and health workers have to be ready to deal with this.

The link between intersectoral collaboration and equity

Some commentators stress the importance of the links between intersectoral collaboration and the equity dimension of PHC. The countries of China and Sri Lanka and the state of Kerala in India are held up as examples of poor countries which have achieved remarkable improvements in the health of their citizens by combining the strategies of equity and an intersectoral approach. Increased access to health services for the population has been accompanied by strategies in other health-related sectors, including

> the entitlement to adequate food; basic education and knowledge which enhanced capacity to cope with health problems, particularly the capacity of females to cope with maternity and child care; and a well-distributed social infrastructure leading to improved housing, water, sanitation and transportation facilities (WHO, 1986a: 27).

The same commentators acknowledge the link also with participation. In all three societies mentioned, there are decentralised structures which allow a voice to people in the community, ensuring that the state has to respond to the expression of community needs (*ibid*: 30). So, we see how, although it may be necessary to distinguish between the three characteristics of a more appropriate health care approach – participation, equity and intersectoral collaboration – this division is simply to help clarify these dimensions. In practice, they should go together. What is perhaps most remarkable in all three countries offered as examples is the similarity in the matter of female education. Access to education has been a major commitment of the state: 'In all three cases, there was a very high level of female participation in the school system. In China, female participation in primary education was 97 per cent in 1982; in Sri Lanka, it was 101 per cent. According to data available for 1978 for Kerala, the rate was 86 per cent as against 55 per cent for the whole of India (*ibid:* 30).

The health worker, who, wherever she or he works, is formed by the medical model but begins to realise its limitations, who seeks to combine the micro and the macro perspectives, and who begins to see health as part of the overall development of individuals and communities, is faced with the challenge of the demands of intersectoral collaboration. The PHC approach calls upon every health worker, at whatever level she or he operates, to acknowledge the contribution of other sectors to the health of individuals and communities and to plan together with them.

Chapter Seven

The Third Pillar: Equity

The demand for a more equitable form of health care is perhaps the most revolutionary of the demands of PHC. Sceptics would say also that it is the least likely to be met. There is a certain amount of ambiguity concerning the possible differences between the terms 'inequality' and 'inequity'. Although clarity is important, it is perhaps enough for present purposes to accept that the term 'inequity' has a moral dimension, suggesting that what is being talked about are avoidable and unjust dimensions of unequal distribution of health resources and disparities in health status. It is clear, of course, that differences will always remain: 'We will never be able to achieve a situation where everyone in the population has the same level of health, suffers the same type and degree of illness and dies after exactly the same life span' (Whitehead, 1991: 219).

These inevitable differences, for example, those caused by biological processes such as ageing, cannot be considered as iniquitous. The equity dimension of PHC concerns those differences in health status and access to health care which are within human control. The concern with equity goes beyond policy statements about equality, stating that all people have an equal right to health and to health care; to make equity an aim means accepting that at present there are severe avoidable imbalances and therefore injustices between people and groups in communities which must be addressed. The Primary Health Care approach incorporates an active concern for justice and the redressing of the balance of health resources. Once again we see that comprehensive PHC poses a real challenge: it does not allow a merely technical approach to health care, it obliges health workers to take a position on the distribution of health resources. The PHC approach acknowledges that certain issues raised by health care are political issues. The organisation of health care involves decisions concerning resource allocation and this puts it squarely in the political domain.

Existing inequalities in health and in health-care provision clearly mirror the pattern of inequalities in the social and economic world; the poorer you are, the more likely you are to be unhealthy (Wilkinson, 1991, 1992), or at least, vulnerable to disease. This being the case, the endorsement of a policy of equity commits health services to a strategy of 'subsidising the disadvantaged' (Gilson, 1989: 325).

The Conference of Alma Ata begins with a denunciation of the existing inequalities in health 'between and within nations'; such disparities in health status and access to health care are unacceptable: 'The existing gross inequality in the health status of the people particularly between developed and developing countries as well as within countries is politically, socially and economically unacceptable and is, therefore, of common concern to all countries' (Alma Ata Declaration I). *Between* nations there is clearly inequality in health. In industrialised countries infant mortality figures are muich lower and people tend to live much longer lives than in the countries of Asia, Africa and Latin America.

The under-five mortality rate in 1989 in Mozambique was 297 per thousand live births; in Japan it was six; in Afghanistan it was 296 and in Sweden seven. In Angola it was 292 and in Finland seven. As we move towards the twenty-first century, life expectancy in these countries is 47 for Mozambique, 79 for Japan; 42 for Afghanistan, 77 for Sweden; 45 for Angola and 75 for Finland (UNICEF, 1991: 102–3). The GNP per capita in Mozambique is $100 and in Japan $21,020 (*ibid*). As a document from WHO, quoting the World Bank, puts it:

> There is no doubt that low per capita income is strongly associated with poor health indicators. Of 42 countries with an infant mortality rate of over 100 per 1000 live births, 26 have per capita incomes below US$400, 9 have per capita incomes between US$400 and US$670, and only a very few have per capita incomes above US$800 (WHO, 1986a: 24).

Of course, people do not have uniform health status in any of these countries; there are differences between groups of people within the same country. The PHC approach as expressed at Alma Ata declares that these inequalities of health states *within* countries are also unacceptable.

There is a noticeable difference in some countries between the health status of the rural and the urban population. In India in

1980 the urban infant mortality rate per 1000 live births was 65 and the rural 124; in Papua New Guinea 50 and 80, respectively (World Development Report, World Bank, in WHO, 1986: 24). Even these statistics are too broad to reveal the true picture of health within urban areas: life for the poor in the urban areas can be worse than that of rural people. A survey in Dakar in Senegal showed that a third of the peri-urban population (often this is a euphemism for slum dwellers) had ascaris, whereas there were only three cases in 400 of the rural population; in the slums of Abidjan, the capital city of Cote d'Ivoire, TB was found to be six times as prevalent as in rural areas of the country. These are some of the findings of the 1990 *Human Development Report* of the United Nations Development Programme (UNDP, 1990: 87) and the same report goes on to document the appalling conditions of the poor in urban situations of the Third World: 'Calcutta, India. Some 3 million people live in shanty towns and refugee settlements without potable water. They endure serious annual flooding and have no way to dispose of refuse or human water ... In Kumasi, Ghana, three of every four households have only one room to live in' (*ibid*: 87–88).

Of course, there are those who say that the health sector has little to do with all of these inequalities: since they are but reflections of the society at large the remedy is to make the world a more just place and inequalities in health status will disappear. In some ways the logic of this argument is inescapable and certainly there is evidence of the fundamental truth that as you improve the general well-being of communities the vital statistics of the population will improve also. The inverse is, of course, also true: the exclusion of groups of people from the possibility of a decent standard of living is at the same time an exclusion from a healthy life. Whether or not the health worker takes the position that she or he can do nothing with this knowledge (that social or material deprivation or satisfaction affect your health), it seems vital at the very least to acknowledge that such linkages exist. Without the understanding of the links between inequalities and ill-health, the danger of inappropriate interventions must be that much greater. What is especially alarming is the growing prosperity gap in most countries between the haves and the have-nots and the parallel gap in health status. Wisner gives the example from Kenya where there have been attempts, as in many countries, to bring down the high rate of infant mortality but where growing social inequalities make this an ever more difficult task: '30,000 families (1 per cent of the population) were enriched and earned, by the early 1970s, more than 1,000 Kenyan pounds a year, while nearly 1.5 million households (63 per cent) made less than 60 pounds a year ... The lack of progress in bringing down infant mortality, then, can hardly be a surprise' (Wisner, 1988: 69).

A strong relationship between social class and health status can be observed throughout the world. Mitchell, among others, draws attention to the difference in health status in Britain between the classes, with levels of chronic depression among working-class women five times greater than that among middle-class women and in general twice the level of chronic illness among people in social class five compared with people in social class one. As she says, 'That's a lot of unnecessary illness we could do without' (Mitchell, 1984: 214). The Black Report of 1980, *Inequalities in Health* (DHSS, 1980) and the debates and studies which have followed it have made it very difficult to deny the links between relative disadvantage and ill-health. The Black Report is based on research in Britain and the pattern it exposes must be true for most industrialised countries. As the four authors of the Black Report, in the foreword to the 1987 document, *The Health Divide*, put it, their research shows that

> material deprivation played the major role in explaining the very unfavourable health record of the poorer sections of the population (especially of the partly skilled and unskilled manual groups making up more than a quarter of the entire population), with biological, cultural and personal lifestyle factors playing a contributory role (Whitehead, 1990: ii).

The inevitable conclusion must be that improvement in the standard of living brings about change in health status: improve or diminish the former and you improve or diminish the latter. However, this sort of analysis, whether in countries like Kenya or Britain can sometimes be used as an excuse for non-activity on the part of health workers: this way of thinking would have it that since health indicators are so closely linked to socio-economic status (this involving in some countries access to land, and in others, as we have seen, poor housing and low income), then there is little that the concerned health worker can do except to work for social structural change. There is another way of looking at the matter: there are many examples from throughout the world of people's struggle against inequalities in health. Health workers committed to 'health for all' can have a certain role in this process. The struggle can be assisted by the systematic examination of the links between social deprivation and social standing in general and the health status of individuals and communities. The denunciation of inequalities in health as being 'politically, socially and economically unacceptable' obliges all health workers to address these issues and to take a position in the face of this struggle. People in disadvantaged groups often need the support of concerned and informed health workers. The acknowledgement of the role of material disadvantage in ill-health also helps prevent the situation of 'blaming the victim' (see also Chapter Eight).

An understanding of the wider causality of ill-health, the move away from a narrow bio-medical view towards a paradigm encompassing a social, cultural and economic causality of health and disease can dispose health workers to recognise and support people's struggle for health. To acknowledge and support such struggles would seem entirely consistent with the PHC approach, embracing as it does the call for equity and people's participation. One can understand that such perspectives might well provide too demanding a challenge to the health worker. The engineering model of health care can allow the health worker to stay within the confines of health care institutions of treatment and the relatively safe view of the biological parameters of disease; the perspectives encouraged by Alma Ata oblige the health worker to step out into the world of unequal resources, relative deprivation and politics. Who could blame the doctors and other health workers who stay within the medical model? In Third World countries where landlessness and exploitative wages are major problems and in industrialised countries where unemployment, dampness and poor housing clearly impact on health, the health workers may not have all the answers to health problems arising from these conditions. But if they are aware of the broader issues and wider causality of ill-health (the 'outer circles') there is less chance of them making the situation worse by haranguing the deprived for their condition of ill-health. This perspective, as we have seen, also predisposes them to be ready to work with other sectors which are engaged in the improvement in the quality of life of disadvantaged people – an orientation towards intersectoral collaboration.

The global dimensions of the problems of inequalities in health have to be understood in the context of the pattern of economic relationships between and within countries. Even some countries where some advances in health status have been achieved are suffering from international monetary pressures in ways which affect the health of the most vulnerable groups within those countries. The financing of the health services in many developing countries has been severely constrained by their burden of debt-servicing. Encouraged to borrow at a time of low interest, developing countries now find themselves in intolerable positions of debt repayment now that the interest rates have risen dramatically. The proportion of export earnings needed simply to service the debt rose sharply in the 1980s (WHO, 1986a: 48). Many countries find that they cannot begin to meet these repayments. 'Structural adjustment' policies have been imposed on them and as a result essential foods have gone up in price and, of course, it is the poor within these countries who suffer the most. For populations struggling to survive, 'structural adjustment' must mean adjustment to increased vulnerability towards disease and premature, preventable death.

Even in simple terms of loss of purchasing power, as Abel-Smith points out, the lack of funds to import drugs has had a disastrous impact on the health services of many developing countries, and again, on account of relative disadvantage within countries, it is often the rural and peri-urban poor who suffer most. He quotes the chairman of the OECD Development Assistance Committee as saying that this situation has led to the disintegration of rural health services, and, by implication also, of services for the urban poor (Abel-Smith, 1986).

It is important to repeat that it is the rural and peri-urban poor who stand to suffer the most in any cuts to the health services in developing and developed countries. Subscribing to equity as a legitimate and necessary concern of the health profession involves giving consideration to the claim that 'inequality is bad for your health' (Wilkinson, 1991). As was said in Chapter Three, the links between poverty and ill-health are well-documented (Townsend and Davidson, 1982). In the early 1990s an editorial in the British Medical Journal reminded us, 'Eliminate poverty and health improves, everyone acknowledges that as a truth for the inhabitants of Third World shanty towns. What recent research in social medicine has now shown is that health continues to improve progressively as people get wealthier' (British Medical Journal, 1990).

In the end, disadvantage in terms of access to health care is consequent on one's socio-economic standing, class and geographical location. It seems to be a hard lesson for health workers to learn that socio-economic status is a major contributory factor to a person's health status and certainly to their access to health care; it seems even harder to incorporate these perceptions into policy and programmes. If we are to make sense at all of the slogan of 'health for all', the rhetoric must be translated into practice and this will sometimes mean a reallocation of health resources away from those most vocal in the articulation of their needs, often the urban middle-class. Such a reallocation requires, of course, a political option, the 'political will' that is often referred to in this context; but it also calls for commitment and dedication on the part of the health profession and even what has been called 'class suicide', since most health workers belong to the class which would have to relinquish some of their relative advantage in any revised sharing out of health resources.

But, of course, it is not only urban middle-class people in general who stand to profit from the continuation of the existing state of inequity which WHO denounces as 'unacceptable'. In many situations throughout the world, health-care provision reflects also the inequalities between men and women. This is surely hardly in dispute: men tend to hold power in society and to profit from whatever social arrangements there are. This includes access to health care. Despite this, women seem to live longer than men in many societies. In Britain, life-expectancy estimates in the early 1980s showed that new-born female children could expect to live six years longer than new-born male children (77 and 71 years, respectively); yet the pattern was reversed concerning morbidity: women had higher levels of acute and chronic illness (Whitehead, 1990). The longer life-span of women is often attributed to such factors as a 'greater natural resistance' to infections and malnutrition (ie women are stronger than men) (WHO, 1986a: 40), but it is also acknowledged that women suffer from high risk of morbidity and mortality in early childhood and their reproductive years: 'This reflects, on the one hand, the low value placed on female children in some societies, and on the other, the high maternal mortality due to lack of maternity and family planning care. Both these situations reflect the low status of women in society' (ibid: 41).

That the health system is male-dominated can hardly be in dispute: in most countries men have most of the powerful and prestigious jobs. Nursing was often considered to be a suitable career for a woman interested in health care: a chance for her to exercise her maternal instincts for the good of sick people at low cost and with no real decision-making as a health-care provider. Women's health has been in the hands of men (Ehrenreich and English, 1978). The women's movement in health care has offered us an example of people's struggle for greater equality in health and has often provided us with examples of demonstrations of male refusal to relinquish medical power.

And again, it would be foolish to suggest that all women suffer equally from discrimination towards them or from male dominance in society or in access to health care. In Western societies, poor black women are much more likely to be more disadvantaged, not just than poor white men, but also than poor white women. Racism in health care is a part of the pattern of inequalities in health and health care in many societies in the West. And of course, although black people in the middle classes may escape from some experiences of racism, since the phenomenon is endemic in Western societies, no black person (and by this I mean no non-white person) will escape fully from its effects. Racism is overt in some societies, like South Africa, where the indigenous population has long been denied access to the same health facilities as the settler white population. In other societies it is, perhaps, more covert: in Britain and the United States, to give but one example, the black population, specifically, those of Afro-Caribbean origin are more at risk of sickle-cell anaemia than whites. This is a painful condition and was, for a long time, largely ignored by the health system. If the white population was prone to this debilitating disease, there would surely have been a greater effort to manage the condition. As it is, black people in the United States and in Britain have been largely responsible for drawing the attention of the health services to the needs of those who suffer from sickle-cell anaemia (Bryan et al, 1985; Brent Community Health Council, 1981).

That there are levels of disadvantage in terms of access to health services there can be no doubt, if one listens to those likely to know. Bryan and her colleagues tell us about the experience of black women in the National Health Service:

> When we approach the Health Service, as clients, we are confronted with a set-up which is both directed and controlled by white, middle-class men. This means that we can expect to face a barrage of assumptions about our race, class and sex by a profession which has no interest in the maintenance of our good health, and little genuine insight into the factors in our lives which cause us to fall ill (Bryan et al, 1985: 90).

These comments from black women in European society draw attention to several of the inequalities underlying health services in many countries: those responsible for the policy and planning of the health services often think they are neutral, serving the interests of all. Such is not the experience of many on the 'other side of the counter', the patients. Doctors and other health workers sometimes call into question the allegation that the medical service can perpetuate injustices in society. To discover what is black women's experience of health services one would have to ask them. Sanders talks of racism within health services which mirrors the racism in society at large. He also gives the example of the use of Depro-Provera as illustrating racism in health care:

> The injectable contraceptive Depro-Provera (DP) has been widely dumped in the Third World, because it is well-established that it has a number of dangerous and unpleasant side-effects. But it is also used on black women in the developed countries. For example, in 1977 in the London Hospital, Whitechapel, two-thirds of the women given DP were Asians (Sanders, 1985: 128.

Again, the cultivated impression of health-care services is that they are somehow above any even covert racial discrimination. The Black Report in Britain, on inequalities in health, highlights the inequalities between social classes; it mentions but does not develop the inequalities between health services for white and black sections of the community. Whitehead laments the lack of studies of black people's experience of the health services and quotes the study of psychiatric hospital patients by Littlewood and Cross which found that 'black patients tended to receive harsher forms of treatment (such as electroconvulsive therapy) than their white counterparts with similar ailments' (Whitehead, 1990: 269). As Whitehead herself suggests, it is to the black community that we must turn for studies of such injustices. A concern for equity would involve the promotion of such studies and discussion of their findings.

Equity and the medical model

The engineering model of health effectively removes the health worker from the dimension of equity and health. By concentrating on the clinical aspects of disease, by promoting the idea that ill-health is mostly a technical and not a social problem, doctors and other health workers are thereby, perhaps sometimes unwittingly, making life easier for themselves. They can attempt to see themselves as the scientists or technicians with the task of putting right the damaged people who arrive on their professional doorsteps. Matters of social and material deprivation and their impact on ill-health can be relegated to the sphere of personal morality rather than professional concern, to charity or social workers.

The health worker who takes seriously the importance of PHC and its demand for greater equity, even in simple terms of access to health care, is in a difficult position, since she or he is in one real sense a part of the problem: not only are the decision-makers and influential leaders from within the profession by definition from the top social classes, but 'doing well' in the profession, developing one's career in the area of a specialisation, removes them in physical and other terms from deprivation and its manifestations. The medical model, as we have seen in Chapter Two, tends by the weight of its own in-built inclination, towards costly institutions of curative care, specialising in the repair of malfunctioning human beings, staffed by costly personnel and mostly based in towns. This is true everywhere, since medical culture is universal, but its effects are more starkly obvious in poor countries:

> 'In Third World countries it is usual for 90 per cent of all in-patients in such institutions (national referral centres) to be drawn from the city in which it is located' (WHO Background paper to the Conference on the Role of Hospitals in PHC, in Paine et al, 1988: 18).

In this regard, the conclusions of an evaluation of medical coverage in Peru reflect the situation in many countries: the bulk of medical personnel are almost inevitably found in urban institutions like hospitals, leaving a large part of the population beyond the reach both of medical personnel and hospital facilities (Zschock, 1989: 331). The report goes on to say that, despite global understanding about the importance of deploying appropriate health personnel nearer the community, physicians (based in such urban institutions) 'accounted for over half of Peru's current health expenditures' (*ibid*). There are, of course, exceptions: Tanzania has, according to the UNDP, 'a fairly good geographical distribution of social services, even with its low income' (UNDP, 1990: 30).

Almost inevitably, of the 90 per cent of the patients in the tertiary hospital referred to above, most will be from the already more affluent areas of the town, especially in countries where hospital fees are levied. So, although urban facilities are catering for only a small proportion of the population, it goes without saying that even this proportion is not usually from the more deprived sections of the community (Harpham et al, 1988). Speaking of Africa as a whole, one report claims that 'more than half of the population has no access to public health services' (UNDP, 1991: 36). In many countries of the world it is indeed the case that there is 'health for the few and those few are the rich'. 'Health for all' as a slogan has been derided for its simplicity, not to say naïvety; perhaps it should rather be applauded for calling to our attention the extent of the distortion of our health services and just how far we are from any such ideal.

It has already been said that most decision-makers in health services are by definition from the middle-class. Doctors, and to a lesser extent, nurses, may find it hard to carry the demand of equity into their professional practice. Whitehead quotes some research from Britain which shows that some general practitioners give shorter consultations to lower-class patients and refer them less frequently to specialist services (Whitehead 1991). She goes on to suggest how such disparities can be tackled: 'Only by monitoring acceptability with the users of services will defects of this nature be revealed. Steps can then be taken to make such services more user friendly' (ibid, 222). Monitoring acceptability with the users, to make services more user-friendly would have to involve more than asking people if they were satisfied with the service given: the link with the promotion of participation is evident here. If people are unaccustomed to see themselves in any position of power, of having rights as well as duties with regards to health care, they are unlikely even to be able to question the acceptability of services. The link with health education is also apparent here, since, as we will see, one sort of health education would concern itself mainly with passing on as efficiently as possible certain medico-technical information. Another sort, more consistent with the participatory ideals of PHC, would be concerned with the declaration of people's rights as much as with their duties. The situation of severe inequalities in health in many parts of the world and for many groups of people highlights the richness of the expression 'empowerment education for health' to which we will return in Chapter Eight.

The privatisation of medical practice is consistent with the professional ethos and image cultivated by the engineering model of health. Doctors are highly trained medical specialists with many years of training behind them. It seems just that they not only get well rewarded even for any public services they perform (for example, for the National Health Service in Britain), but that they are able to charge high fees for private practice. The commercialisation of the treatment of ill-health – for that is what we are talking about – reinforces the medical model: doctor as the source of specialised technical information, patients as uninformed laypeople in need of this professional wisdom; doctor and his skills as expensive commodities, patients as consumers, both of the doctor's time and skills and of the prescription of pharmaceuticals to which he holds the key, if they can afford the cost. All of this does little to encourage any move towards the ideal of health as 'people's business' let alone health care as 'free to all at the point of need'. What we seem to be moving towards is a monopoly of necessary commodities which, like petrol, are not likely to become accessible to all. Another point to remember in the discussion about private practice and the general high cost of medical care is the peculiar contradiction, again more acute in Third World countries, that the expensive commodity which is the doctor has often been trained, at least to some extent, at public expense. Trained to serve the community would surely be acceptable, but trained to practise private medicine on behalf of those who can afford his services in urban settings is quite another matter.

What of the commercialisation of medical skills in the Third World? Many rural areas were already without doctors in any case, but even in the poorest countries there seems to be a worrying trend (at least in terms of a move away from any policies of equity) to promote the idea that people do not appreciate what they do not pay for. In times of economic difficulties, UNDP says, 'government officials (often with foreign donors) are turning to local people for voluntary contributions to maintaining local services. In such self-help schemes, villagers offer their free labour for construction and maintenance work, contribute food for government personnel and pay for drugs and other services' (UNDP, 1990: 74). The 'voluntary' nature of these contributions is questionable, especially when we are talking about the purchase of drugs and the move towards 'community financing'. As has been said many times, the 'willingness to pay does not imply ability to pay' (Gilson, 1988: 78). As one commentator on the 'Bamako Initiative', a scheme to ensure the financing of PHC through the use of a revolving drug fund and decentralised management, says, the danger is that once again, the poorest of the poor are always the ones who suffer from any increased commercialisation of medical care (Kanji, 1989).

The equity dimension means a fresh look at those who might be disadvantaged in terms of health care and in that group must surely feature disabled people. The 'medical' approach to disability was often to hospitalise and treat where possible. Present moves towards rehabilitation and the management of disability in the community with the maximum control being exercised by disabled people themselves do not fit easily into the medical model. The community rehabilitation approach seeks to place the matter of rehabilitation in the social context and looks much more to the amelioration of the handicapping environment in which disabled people live than to the removal of disabled people from the community:

> Social integration is viewed as active participation of disabled and handicapped persons in the mainstream of community life. In order to achieve this aim it is necessary to provide adequate rehabilitation for all the disabled and handicapped and to reduce to a minimum all handicapping conditions in all aspects of their environment (WHO, 1981: 10).

'Adequate rehabilitation' cannot be taken to mean some cheap alternative to institutionalised care. One has, yet again, to be as aware of the abuse of a progressive vocabulary to mask lack of concern or care as colonised marginalised Africans had to be of the exhortations by colonial officers that they should be 'self-reliant'.

Genuine community rehabilitation seems much closer to the spirit of PHC than to the forms of institutionalised care previously deemed appropriate for disabled people. David Werner, one of the great promoters of PHC, in his introduction to his book on rehabilitation, places the integration of disabled people into society firmly on the plane of equity and social justice when he says that too much emphasis and too little thought have gone into trying to make disabled people 'normal' in a society which has very dubious claims to that description itself:

> Too often 'normal' in our society is selfish, greedy, narrow-minded, prejudiced – and cruel to those who are weaker or different from others. We live in a world where too often it is 'normal' and acceptable for the rich to live at the expense of the poor, and for health professionals to earn many times the wages of those who produce their food but cannot afford their services ... This large book, then, is a small tool in the struggle not only for the liberation of the disabled, but for their solidarity in the larger effort to create a world where more value is placed

on being human than on being 'normal' (Werner, 1987: A4).

Primary Health Care and equity

Equity and intersectoral collaboration are two of the three pillars of the PHC approach; they go together: if one accepts a broad causality of disease one is open to the possibility that housing, for example, plays an important part in the maintenance of health. This was understood in Europe in the earlier part of the twentieth century when communities were threatened with TB. The lessons, unfortunately, seem to get forgotten too quickly. The engineering model of health, as we have said, easily draws the attention away from the wider circles of disease causality and health enhancement, away from the macroscope. The Edinburgh Research Unit in Health and Behavioural Change (RUHBC, 1989: 104) documents studies which show that improvement in housing has brought improvement in health conditions; the same Unit highlights the research of Martin (1987) into the health hazards of living in damp houses, a condition all too common in more deprived parts of Britain as well as in many situations of the Third World. Taking these studies seriously obliges health workers to be interested in the work of sectors which impact on health, like housing. Any professional body, or people's group which is in the business of promoting better (in the sense of healthier) housing, would be justified in looking for support from health workers with a PHC approach.

Unfortunately, such support is not always forthcoming. From a medical as opposed to health perspective, it is possible to say that conditions of inequality are no concern of the health profession, even though they impact on people's health in very important ways. The present medical orientation of health workers tends to produce disease-oriented health workers. Community development workers like those supporting people's actions for improvements in living conditions such as housing to make them more health-enhancing would have a better claim to being health workers (Jones, 1983). The PHC message is that an equity orientation means that there must be at least some intersectoral planning and collaboration, in this case between medicine and those involved in housing. This statement has universal validity. PHC points the way towards a more adequate health care system in any society. Its three pillars are just as important in Glasgow,

Scotland and Washington, DC as they are, for example, in the towns and countryside of China.

Not all that goes under the name of PHC is necessarily at the forefront of the struggle against inequity in society. Many so-called PHC programmes, for example, are 'aimed' at women, yet whether their impact on the lives of the women is always liberating is not so clear. Sometimes their effect is to add to the already heavy burden a woman already carries in caring for the health of families (MacCormack, 1989).

The struggle for justice in health

The acknowledgement of the importance of intersectoral collaboration, people's participation and the equity dimension of health-care provision guarantees a more difficult life for the health worker. First of all, he/she must try to build in such preoccupations to their professional practice. But what of activities outside the health sector? In the matter of equity, what must be the response of the health worker to people's struggle for justice in health care provision? What about people's struggle for better housing, or for more access to land to grow food for their families? Of course, no one should dare to tell all health workers to be ready to risk imprisonment for supporting such struggles, which would be the case in some countries. But within the room for manoeuvre open to each individual the PHC approach definitely encourages the idea that health workers are on the side of people's struggle for health.

A seminar of health activists in Latin America in 1988 discussed the document of Alma Ata and spoke out in favour of the document's commitment to equity. For the strategies of Alma Ata to become a reality, however, the health workers pointed out that 'primary health care can only emerge from a spirit of justice and social equity'. But they sound a note of warning also and raise some doubts about certain aspects of the Alma Ata document. We have to realise, they say,

> the magnitude of the opposition coming from the dominant sectors ... From this perspective our doubts about the Alma Ata contents are valid. Have they constituted a strategy for change in the sense of our people's liberation, the dignity of human beings and the improvement in the quality of life? Or has this strategy become an instrument used by the dominant sectors to

promote their interests? (Popular Education and Primary Health Care Network, 1989).

It has to be remembered that these doubts about the vision of PHC put forward by Alma Ata come from a network of educationists and health workers in Latin America committed to many of the principles of the PHC approach: they looked at the Alma Ata strategy and, while endorsing its principles, have question marks about whether it goes far enough in the active promotion of justice in health matters. It would be a wonderful challenge to all groups of health workers to examine their own policies and practice in the light of Alma Ata and its strategies. Would doctors, nurses and other health workers in North America, Europe and other continents find, after such an examination, that their practice left Alma Ata behind?

Chapter Eight

Education for Health: Lifestyle Education or Life-context Education?

In theory, education for health, or health education, is an important component of most health services. Increasingly, health programmes have an educational component or a health education division – this more recently replaced by a division of health promotion. In earlier chapters it has been said that the dominant medical model is an engineering one and its non-participatory ethos makes it difficult for health professionals to work *with* rather than *for* communities. A model of professional practice in which the professional is the active agent (the doctor) and the client passive (the patient) does not lend itself easily to participatory planning practices. When compliance is the attitude and response expected of the patient it is hard to envisage much scope for participation. The PHC approach is part of the search for a new model of health care. The approach calls upon health professionals to go beyond the framework of reference supplied by the medical model in which they have been formed. There is, unfortunately, another constraining model, this time an educational one. In other words, in addition to the restrictions imposed by an engineering medical model of health, when health workers take on the role of education they are also often limited by the educational model within which they operate.

The dominant model of education in the world today is one of information transfer in which the teacher possesses the knowledge which he or she then passes on by a variety of means, modern or otherwise, to the learner. The teacher acts, the learner receives. The teacher is in the active role, the learner's rather passive role is to be as receptive as possible. When this model of learning is applied to health education, what we have is the health professional telling and the patient or community listening and learning and doing what is recommended. The health message is a medical message – the medical information necessary to remedy the situation – to be passed on to the recipient in as effective a way as possible. The effectiveness will be measured by the extent to which the learner implements the suggested activity. Fortunately or otherwise, the evidence shows that people often do not do what they are told, even when the teller is as prestigious a person as a doctor.

There seems to be a remarkably simplistic notion of health education in the minds of many health workers which confuses health information with health education. Of course, there are many health workers who go far beyond the simple transfer of knowledge when they take on the role of educator or health communicator. Nevertheless, what the public are faced with in most encounters with the health profession is a professional trained in the engineering model of health care and when that health worker becomes 'educator' the assumption is often that he or she is someone with the technical health knowledge which the less-informed person, the patient, needs. The task is to transmit this knowledge. Many health workers seem to think that if you tell people what to do then they will do it. The AIDS epidemic offers a clear example of what many in the medical profession believe about education: one gets told on numerous occasions by health workers, tell people that AIDS is a virus, how it is transmitted and how dangerous it is and they will change their behaviour. Many AIDS 'education' programmes are based on just such shaky pedagogical foundations. This is because this is the way in which much health education has happened. Tell women that unhygienic conditions contaminate food, so they should wash their hands, that smoking is bad for you and should be stopped, that brown bread or protein-enriched cassava is good for you and should be eaten instead of what you are eating now, that diarrhoea causes dehydration and should be dealt with by oral rehydration therapy (ORT): health education becomes a series of messages to be transmitted to the public by the knowledgeable professional. The public's role in this encounter is to listen carefully, understand the message and carry out the instructions: to do what they are told.

The Edinburgh Research Unit in Health and Behavioural Change describes the three underlying assumptions of most health education programmes as the following: that human beings are primarily rational beings, that if they are given the correct information about changed behaviour being desirable, they will follow it and that this change can be brought about without undue consideration of the context. As the same researchers go on to say, however, 'Neither experience, history nor experiment supports these premises' (RUHBC, 1989: 67). In other words, there are a lot of unsuccessful or dubiously successful health education programmes. Because human beings are more than disembodied minds, information about behaviour, on its own, however 'correct' or 'desirable' in the eyes of the professional, is often not perceived as being preferable behaviour by the receiver, and the context in which the receiver lives and is expected to implement the good advice given has an enormous influence on whether or not it gets translated into practice. Much health education is only about behaviour and ignores context.

The model of education underlying many health education programmes closely parallels the medical engineering model; the two types of professional behaviour engendered by each model reinforce one another. In medicine the doctor is active and the power in the diagnosis of what is to be remedied lies with him; the patient is passive and acted upon. Many people's experience of education is of a similar mode of interaction: the teacher is active and the learner is passive. 'Success' lies in remembering, repeating and in doing what you have been told.

Education for behavioural change or for empowerment?

Perhaps the most influential theory of health education in Western health services over the last two decades has been the health belief model (Becker, 1974, Janz and Becker, 1984). This model – a framework both for understanding the process of people's acceptance of health messages and for planning such interventions – is based on the hypothesis that behavioural change depends on two main variables: the value which an individual places on a particular goal and the individual's estimation of the likelihood that a given action will achieve that goal (Janz and Becker, 1984: 2). The individual's perception of the severity of – and his/her own susceptibility to – a particular disease will influence their response to health education. Another major influencing factor will be their perceptions of the benefits to be gained by changing behaviour and the obstacles that would need to be overcome for them to adopt this behavioural change. Some emphasis is put by those advocating this framework on 'cues to action': the presence or absence of stimuli to change. More recently, health educators have been encouraged to adopt an 'expanded health belief model', expanded to incorporate the notion of 'self-efficacy' (Rosenstock et al, 1988). This notion is drawn from the work of social (or 'cognitive') learning theorists like Bandura (Bandura, 1977a and 1977b) and suggests that another important factor to be considered when planning health education is the individual's perception of his/her ability to do what is being asked. As applied, for example, to the question of smoking, this expanded health belief model (HBM) would make the following prediction: 'In order, say, for a woman ... to quit smoking (BEHAVIOUR) for health reasons (OUTCOME), she must believe both that cessation will benefit her health (OUTCOME EXPECTATION) and also that she is capable of quitting (EFFICACY EXPECTATION) (Rosenstock et al, 1988: 178).

Another related model often referred to is the PRECEDE model proposed by Green (Green et al, 1980). Its purpose is to help health educators to diagnose the health problem to be tackled; its main tools are the analyses of 'predisposing and reinforcing factors' which will enhance the likelihood of behavioural change. In some ways the PRECEDE model can be seen as complementary to the health belief model, since the factors Green and his colleagues speak about are factors which influence the values and judgements which are the focus of the health belief model. Some consideration is given to the context of the learner in so far as it is acknowledged that this context will help or hinder the acceptance of the suggested change.

With the appearance of AIDS on the international health scene there has been a growth of interest in what has been called 'protection motivation theory' (Prentice-Dunn et al, 1986), linked again to the preceding models by its emphasis on individuals' perceived susceptibility to disease; the emphasis here is on how motivated or otherwise individuals are to protect themselves. This leads to a consideration of the effects of fear arousal on health behaviour. In other words, sometimes fear of the consequences of unchanged behaviour can motivate the learner to accept the health education message.

The health belief model and other, related approaches to health education have been called the preventive model of health education (Tones et al, 1990). It can be seen that the main discipline which has contributed to this framework is psychology. Psychology, by definition, focuses on the working of individual cognition and motivation. The medical model also, as we have noted, is focused particularly on the individual. The health belief model has been criticised, among other things, for this narrow focus, suggesting that individual human beings function in a sort of social isolation. Despite a move towards recognition of the social and cultural variables in health education approaches (Azjen and Fishbein, 1980), from psychologically oriented models to socio-psychological models, some critics, like Bunton and his colleagues (Bunton et al, 1991) suggest that the health belief model still puts 'too great an emphasis on the use of psychologically oriented models' while failing to fully draw upon relevant social theory. They also draw attention to the individualist focus of these models: 'There has been a tendency to present a rather simplified picture of social structure and process whilst focusing mainly on individual aspects of change' (Bunton et al, 1991: 155). The assumption behind health education based on the HBM kind is that people have the means and possibility of implementing changes in their lives. It has been pointed out that sometimes people are simply not in a position to carry out the good advice they are given. The circumstance in which they live limit their possible choices of action. Moran puts it clearly when he says that health education 'has placed its major emphasis on achieving voluntary changes in individual behaviour through expert interventions which, while purportedly politically neutral, neglect the wider social and economic forces affecting health over which isolated individuals have little or no control' (Moran, 1986: 122).

The Edinburgh Research Unit for Health and Behavioural Change also points out the limitations of the individualist perspective of the health belief model; this and the notions of perceived susceptibility and severity can be seen as fitting 'well with an allopathic medical paradigm' (RUHBC, 1989: 9). These researchers draw attention to the fact that the model focuses on the negative aspects of health belief, a point which could be made of Green's PRECEDE model also. Green's model is, in fact, called a 'diagnostic' approach. We have already pointed out the pathologising perspective contained in the notion of diagnosis. The diagnosis, the search for what is wrong, is focused on the individual, rarely on the wider negative influences on health of economy and social environment. The diagnostic approach is a microscopic rather than a macroscopic view. Moreover, with such an orientation, the focus is not going to be on what there is in the individual or community which is health-enhancing, health-promoting. If we go back to our example of the traditional birth attendants (TBAs) and think in terms of using the health belief model as a framework for constructing a health education programme we run into problems.

If we focus only on the severity and susceptibility of the dimensions of diseases which can result from potential 'at risk' behaviour of the TBAs, in the way encouraged by the model, perhaps with a little 'fear arousal' by stressing the risk of death from such conditions as neonatal tetanus, we might successfully avoid disease. But this would surely be only part of our educational objective. We would have missed the opportunity to build on the strengths of the TBAs and encourage their work of providing support for mothers. From this we can see that health education often consists of health information selected on the basis of eliminating what is defective in people's behaviour rather than in building their confidence in their ability to construct a healthier life. It is education or training for behaviour modification rather than education for empowerment.

On the social dimension of learning, Bunton et al. say that 'individual elements of belief, value, attitude and intention exist and are constructed, maintained or changed in interaction with the social environment, through special interaction ... In other words, the context of behaviour – the social setting in which attitudes, values and beliefs are constructed – is central to any account of behavioural change' (*ibid:* 156). They go on to say that there is a need for a shift in focus from that on inner states and qualities towards that of collective behaviour in organisational and community settings. They refer to Graham's study of smoking in women (Graham, 1986), which shows that smoking can be a coping strategy: 'clearly behavioural change programmes would need to take account of the material and social circumstances of these women' (Bunton et al, 157). Other researchers point to the need to incorporate the influence of 'significant others' in any health education strategy (Zimmerman et al, 1989), a perspective that would be consistent with a PHC approach to health education, given what we know of the role of groups and community structures in promoting people's participation. All of this suggests a move towards life-context health education. At the moment, there is considerable emphasis in health education upon lifestyles rather than life-context. The medical model reinforces this focus on the individual's behaviour and what he or she should be doing to their own body. It helps remove the focus from other health-threatening dimensions of social existence which could very well be the legitimate object of health education programmes. Many commentators have suggested that the focus of health education on lifestyles, while ignoring the threat to individual and collective health of the environment, should be described as 'victim-blaming': at least implicitly making people – often women as the main health guardians of the families – feel guilty that they are not doing well enough for their families. Ryan (1976) has drawn our attention to the danger of 'victim-blaming' and Crawford (1977, 1988) shows that the individualistic and lifestyle focus of much of health education which has this tendency is often a deflection of attention away from some of the social causes of illness. Fortunately, some people resist this sort of health 'education'. The most vivid illustration of the weakness of lifestyle-focused health education was given to me by some Scottish women who were showing me the dampness of the council houses in which they lived: 'Don't talk to us about brown bread and jogging, here is the cause of bad health in our community' (McCormack, 1991). Some victims refuse to be blamed.

The main point of the criticisms of the preventive model of health education is that the considerable focus on the psychology of individuals in order to persuade them to change their behaviour often does not work, in terms of getting them to change their behaviour. The life-context and its influence on behaviour seems to get ignored and, as a result, people can acknowledge the 'correctness' of health information messages without translating them into action.

A communication strategy which has received much attention in the world of health education in recent years and which many international agencies have endorsed as a useful educational approach is what is known as *social marketing*. There is much to be learned, it is said, from the world of commerce and advertising: commercial companies research a community for ways in which to influence their consumer needs and then use this knowledge to sell their product. Some have encouraged health educators to learn from the commercial world. After all, the argument goes, big business knows how to convince people: why shouldn't health professionals be able to adopt or at least adapt its approach for their own ends? Some would say that the aims of health promotion and of health marketing have much in common. But as Tones and his colleagues point out, 'there is a fundamental difference in the nature of the products on offer'. The commercial world, they say, is intent on gratifying some real or imagined need:

> By contrast, health education is frequently trying to sell a product which commercial advertisers would consider no-one in their right mind would buy! Potential customers are not uncommonly urged to stop doing something they

find enjoyable and start doing something unpleasant or difficult ... the product which is being promoted by health education is frequently intangible and offers gratification in the (often distant) future (Tones et al, 1990: 167–8).

The commercial world, on the other hand, is in the business of offering immediate gratification, for a price, sometimes deferred.

The approach of social marketing may fit well the manipulation of popular choices in tobacco and soft drinks. As a health education approach, however, it has serious deficiencies. It assumes that what is called for is the adoption of a technical solution to the disease problem and the means of transferring the minimal necessary 'message' involved into the lives of those to be taught. It fits well, too, with the approach of the medical model with its focus on the individual and ignores what we have called the wider circles of causality of ill-health. As Naidoo says, 'Advertising health as a commodity obscures the social construction of health, and it is in this sense that the marketing type of health promotion is individualism in a new guise (Naidoo, 1986: 28). Social marketing can seem like a 'modern' approach to health education; some health-education programme planners have felt that in the door-to-door, person-to-person sales technique of the commercial world, there is a fine example of the 'power of persuasion' and an obviously appropriate educational example. But as Jobert says, in the context of those family-planning programmes in Third World countries which have adopted a marketing approach to education, what we have are 'concepts and action strategies largely borrowed from marketing and management, as if changes in attitude towards birth could be organised using the same criteria as the sale of toothpaste in Iowa' (Jobert, 1985: 18).

The 'social marketing' approach involves, among other things, the use of the mass media to diffuse the message as widely as possible. Television and radio are very attractive to some modern health educators. The work of communicators like McAnay (1980), however, should have warned us against any simplistic faith in the educative power of radio and television in anything except a supportive role, since the evidence he presents is that the one-way nature of these media can result in a wide dissemination of information but on its own is often unlikely to persuade people to change behaviour to which they are accustomed or attached. Despite this, the mass media seem to many in the medical world to be the ideal tool of the health educator. Health information has become confused with health education. This is not to deny that, as part of a strategy of using a multimedia approach, the mass media can have a useful role to play:

> Like television and the print media, radio has the disadvantage of being a one-way medium of communication. This can be partly overcome, however, by organising groups of people who meet regularly to listen to radio programmes, with the help of a trained amateur to stimulate and guide the discussion (O'Sullivan-Ryan et al, undated:10).

The same report gives the example of the programme in India which uses the *anganwadi* or child-care centre as a meeting place for groups of women: the programme supplies the radio and trains the child-care centre staff. It is claimed that every week over 10,000 groups of 10 to 35 Indian women listen to programmes on pregnancy and early childhood. A survey in Tamil Nadu found that nearly half of the women in the listening groups had improved their family diets (*ibid*). A famous pioneering example of this approach was the *Mtu Ni Afya* (The Person is Health) campaign in Tanzania which was part of the drive for universal literacy in that country. The approach was multimedia in the way already described and, apart from anything else, a fine example of intersectoral collaboration: education and health working together (Hall, 1978). There are a considerable number of such multimedia approaches in Latin America: the mass-media, often either radio or cassette player is used to provide a health message input; an organised group listens under the guidance of a trained facilitator and there is printed material for use by both group and facilitator (*ibid*).

The move towards health promotion, as well as the Healthy Cities Movement, which seeks to implement health promotion, can be seen as initiatives in the spirit of Alma Ata which are aimed at improving on traditional health education and as moves away from the influence of the more narrow, individualistic, medical model. Health promotion would include actions and campaigns to create a healthy environment as well as to provide health information and would in principle allow for the tackling of social causes of ill-health as well as their symptoms. Understood in this way, health promotion is a 'mediating strategy between people and their environments', incorporating both personal choice and social responsibility in health (WHO, 1986b: 70). In other words, the health promotion approach goes beyond the classical health education preoccupation with individual behaviour and lifestyles and includes a consideration of the conditions, both social and economic, in which individuals live and which can have an important influence on their health (WHO, 1986c, 1987). Perhaps the most significant difference between health education as generally understood and health promotion is that, whereas much health education tended to focus on the individual and his/her responsibility for their health and considered the context or environment only as factors impinging on individual decisions, health promotion makes the context, physical, economic, cultural and social, legitimate foci of the educational process itself. What is there in your economic or social condition which impinges on your health? This is a legitimate question in the perspective of health promotion, but would not be in most 'classical' health education programmes. Tones et al. define health promotion as 'any combination of education and related legal, fiscal, economic, environmental and organisational interventions designed to facilitate the achievement of health and the prevention of disease' (Tones et al, 1990: 4). This represents a welcome move away from the microscope to the macroscope and can lead to collective lobbying against unhealthy environments. The 'New Public Health' (Ashton et al, 1988) and 'Healthy Cities' initiatives can be seen as public health movements in the spirit of Alma Ata.

The 'Healthy Cities' initiative was launched in 1986 by WHO and the Department of Public Health at Liverpool University. It represents an attempt to put the principles of 'health for all' into practice (Ashton et al, 1986). It was an acknowledgement that by the year 2000 half of the world's population would be living in or around towns. It was also a move away from the individualistic and victim-blaming orientations of much of conventional health education. Ashton, who has done much to develop Healthy Cities, shows that, as a health education movement it builds on work such as that of Dennis who held that health education should have three strands: biological knowledge; consumer information and a concern with the wider issues affecting health. These wider issues must include activities of the 'anti-health' sector of the economy as well as unemployment, schooling, pollution etc. (Ashton et al, 1988: 47). Ashton and Dennis' 'wider issues' would correspond to the 'outer circles of health' we have referred to. Making these an essential focus of health education is clearly moving away from the narrower engineering model of health care, towards a macroscopic perspective.

The Healthy Cities Movement and health promotion in general have emerged from Alma Ata under the general umbrella of the 'health for all' movement. So they are European manifestations of the Primary Health Care approach. Unfortunately, although Alma Ata has clearly been inspirational for these movements, and they have achieved much, their proponents do not speak of themselves or see themselves as promoters of PHC. This may be because they do not like the vocabulary, or because they are not aware of the considerable movement towards a wider vision of health care which PHC represents in the Third World, but there are several unfortunate consequences of this omission.

Firstly, not to acknowledge that Health Cities and the version of health promotion which inspires it are part of the PHC movement inevitably weakens PHC as an international movement working towards a more appropriate health care system. Healthy Cities espouses participation, working with other sectors and the dimension of equity, the three pillars of PHC. PHC workers in the Third World would immediately see the aims and methods of health promotion as belonging to the PHC approach. In the Third World there are many groups and movements working towards the same ends, all acknowledging the PHC banner. The Healthy Cities movement in Europe could learn much from these which have been struggling for a more appropriate health system for at least several decades before the Healthy Cities initiative began. Is the West open to such lessons?

Another unfortunate result of seeing Healthy Cities as something apart from PHC is that this can unwittingly reinforce the medical model, the very opposite, surely, of what is intended by the proponents of the movement. How? Alma Ata and the vision of PHC which it promotes keep together the curative, promotive, educational and rehabilitative dimensions of health care (Alma Ata Declaration, VII, 3). In so doing, PHC is resisting the conceptual and operational separation of treatment and prevention which fits the engineering model of health care, with prestige and often scarce resources going to clinical medicine to the neglect of prevention, promotion and rehabilitation. Of course, operationally, distinctions have to be made but the comprehensive model of PHC of Alma Ata is a challenge to all health workers and programmes, not just to those involved in preventive work. If Healthy Cities is seen as just a campaign of some interested people or disadvantaged groups, its contribution to a better health system is diminished. The more health promotion becomes distinct from the world of curative care, the more this latter is allowed to continue to be seen as the real work of medicine, and consequently, the more the PHC challenge is diluted. Promoters of Healthy

Cities projects who see their relevance for cities of the Third World should see such projects as necessarily linked to the whole organisation of health-service provision and be careful not to drive further apart curative and preventive services in the name of progress.

The medical intervention or engineering model of health care has had a powerful influence on the kind of health education pursued in many countries. The health promotion approach consistent with the comprehensive vision of Alma Ata tends not to fit with the medical model which, in terms of health education, has an affinity with selective versions of PHC. One striking example of the negative influence on education for health of the medical model, especially in combination with an option for selective PHC, can be seen in Bangladesh and the work of the Bangladesh Rural Advancement Committee (BRAC). BRAC is an indigenous non-government organisation in Bangladesh which began as a research organisation dedicated, as its name suggests, to the advancement of the population of the country, with a special concern for the marginalised and less privileged. The organisation produced some excellent work showing the terrible trap of poverty and powerlessness in which millions of Bangladeshi people are caught (BRAC, 1980). The organisation saw itself as an ally of people in the struggle against injustice and their partner in the social development of the country. In the 1970s and early 1980s the group was involved in participatory research: professionals and populations working together in deepening their under-standing of social reality. From this a people-centred education methodology evolved, a methodology which could lead to structural social change; to quote from BRAC itself:

> Previously everyone knew some of the things that were going on because they were right in front of them, but it was a shadowy, partial way. By adding this knowledge to that of others and then by analysing and calculating everything, they could see in a clear open way for the first time, and so realistically consider the possibility of change (BRAC, 1980: 4).

BRAC showed an interest in the perceptions and understanding of poor people and tried to systematically record these as, for example, in their publication, *Peasant Perceptions: Famine* (BRAC, 1979). We can see that BRAC had an educational methodology in place, one geared to working with groups of people for social change, a collective building-up of understanding and confidence, aiming, in the vocabulary of Hope and Timmel, at social transformation (Hope and Timmel, 1984). Such an approach seems to be very far from a narrow focus on behaviour or lifestyles and includes a strong focus on context as influencing behaviour and therefore as constituting a potentially major impediment to progress.

An interest was shown in health and specifically in diarrhoea, seen as a major illness in the lives of many of the population. BRAC has become one of the most prominent promoters of oral rehydration therapy (ORT) (see Chapter Four). Given BRAC's stated understanding of the 'net' of poverty and the need for collective empowering education, one could have hoped that the latter would guide BRAC's approach to the problem of diarrhoea. Surely here, we might think, we will have an example of health education for empowerment.

In fact, what BRAC is doing with ORT is far from this. Women (generally as individuals) are taught the seven 'points' of good diarrhoea management, which include the recognition of the signs of dehydration and the steps to be followed in the administration of oral solution. The teaching method is thought to be appropriate and up-to-date, since it emphasises one-to-one contact between the instructor and the women. The instructor is highly motivated, since she is paid according to the number of points which the mothers taught by her can remember. The emphasis is on a training programme which helps the individual mother retain the main points of the technical information she needs on when and how to administer ORT correctly (Abed, 1983). BRAC has done what many 'experts' recommend and taken from the world of commercial selling the technique of social marketing. Highly motivated door-to-door salespeople succeed in selling commercial goods, so why not specially trained health workers?

By 1986 more than 8 million households had been visited and the mothers in them 'trained' (Chowdhury, 1990). This no doubt represents a major achievement. However, as we have said, here we have an organisation capable of understanding the links between poverty and disease, and therefore of embarking upon programmes of prevention including education and the use of ORT. Its own approach and research provided it with an analysis of powerlessness at the grassroots level, and so a way into understanding the causes of diarrhoeal disease; we have an organisation capable of giving an 'empowering' education, helping people to treat the symptoms of the problem while looking for ways of tackling its causes. But what we actually have is an organisation being seduced instead into the belief that 'social marketing', the almost mechanistic transfer of health information to people, is the answer to health education. Instead of a life-context health education, we have a lifestyle health education. Health education has become confused with health information.

Considerable funds and energy have been spent on this programme. The evaluation of this ORT education, by the Director of BRAC himself, says that the retention level (how much accurate information is remembered) was high even after six months. 'But the utilisation-rate range from different areas varies widely (8–80 per cent) (Abed, 1983: 261). In other words, even in its own terms, there are problems with this approach. Moreover, nothing is said about an examination of the people's problems and perceptions or the possible social and economic dimensions of causes and solutions to the problem; the focus is very clearly on the technical. As we saw in Chapter Four, ORT can have a role as part of the answer to the problems of diarrhoea. As Werner says, it is a 'stop-gap measure' which supposes that the intervention is part of a wider programme of tackling the environmental and social causes of the disease (Werner, 1988). Therefore, although BRAC call this 'empowerment through education' (Chowdhury, 1990), it is hard to see how such an approach merits this title. As an educational methodology it seems almost exactly what Freire denounces as 'banking education'. In some other programmes in the Third World there is also the tendency to confuse information with education, as shown by the type of evaluation which would consider a programme 'successful' if information is retained as in the example given above. At least BRAC had the courage to go beyond the retention rate to look at utilisation, the more difficult but surely more crucial dimension of health education. Of what use is health information if it is not translated into health-enhancing action by people?

Selective Primary Health Care, of which BRAC's ORT programme is a good example, seems to call for a type of education which sees education as information transfer, a series of packaged messages to be delivered to people. BRAC, originally an organisation with deep insights into the powerlessness of poor people, has recently been more involved in the formation of village-health committees and mothers' clubs in order 'to ensure participation and continuity' and this may mean development of their educational methodology along the lines of their original philosophy. It remains to be seen whether any education for comprehensive PHC they embark upon will draw as much support and attention as their selective approach to education for PHC has done.

Towards a comprehensive Primary Health Care approach to health education

The three pillars of the PHC approach are again relevant here. Equity: people have a right of access to useful health information; this may even include information about structures which impede their health; the social status of some people impinges on their health and this is a legitimate focus of 'health education'. Intersectoral collaboration is also important in a PHC approach to health education: health workers who see the importance of education cannot ignore the fact that other sectors – notably education, but others as well – are in the business of educating the public in many health-related matters and have lessons and programmes to share. Participation: top-down, didactic teaching methods are inconsistent with the PHC approach, with its call for genuine participation on the part of individuals and communities in the health-care system.

The matter of participation is of particular importance in any reflection on education and health. We have seen (in Chapter Five) that participation involves the sharing of power: the acceptance by health professionals that the role of the public in interacting with health-care systems is not just one of carrying out duties, but of knowing and exercising their rights as well. Ultimately, the success of a health programme could be measured by the extent to which an individual or a community has achieved autonomy vis-à-vis the health profession. The health worker assumes the role of facilitating this process. It should come as no surprise that the WHO committee working on education in PHC stressed the need for a participation dimension to this education. Historically, the report of the committee concludes, people were not involved in the development of health services; they were, and one can say *are*, 'the passive receivers of a service when it existed'. However, 'many policy-makers and governments have gradually come to understand that men and women ... are capable of being actively involved in matters regarding their own health' (WHO, 1983:39). The process by which policy-makers and governments are coming to an understanding of the need for a more participatory approach to development and to health education may be more gradual than the documents of WHO might suggest, but the call for such participation seems very logical. Once again, we come back to the fundamental question: *is health education a matter of behaviour modification or of empowerment of people?*

Of course, to state the debate in this way does not imply that even those who are concerned with education for health as empowerment are not involved in the matter of behavioural change. There can be little dispute about behaviour modification being an important element in all health education. But prisoners who from one day to the next take exercise when previously they did not, because they are ordered to do so and threatened with punishment if they do not, have indeed modified their behaviour, but could this change be attributed to health education? Communities who dig pit latrines because threatened with fines if they do not, have in one sense modified their behaviour or at least their environment. But if they do not use the latrines or maintain them, then the process of persuading them to dig these facilities can hardly be called health education in any positive sense.

The simple taxonomy of Cohen and Uphoff concerning participation can be useful here: what kind of participation of the public has been demanded in the above examples? Implementation, no doubt: both the prisoners taking exercise and the villagers digging pit latrines were involved in the implementation of the activity concerned. There were public benefits, probably: both groups at least stood to gain potentially from the activities. But participation in evaluation and decision-making which have been described as the kinds of participation which mark out the genuine sort and the kind called for by the PHC approach are both noticeably lacking in our examples. They are also, by and large, missing from most health education programmes.

The WHO committee which saw the need for a participatory dimension to health education, also stressed its intersectoral and equity dimensions:

> No longer is health, or its education component, the prerogative of any single group; it is the concern of all who are involved in cultural and socio-economic development ... Men and women ... are demanding social equity ... It is by respecting the individual's freedom and dignity that health education can provide the setting that will lead to the goal of health for all by the year 2000 (WHO, 1983: 40).

One can comment on the idealism of this approach, but by being consistent with the demands of the three pillars of PHC, this WHO document serves the useful task of offering some criteria for assessing the appropriateness of health education.

Health workers sometimes seem to involve themselves in educational activities without consulting educators; the idea that they may have something to learn about effective and appropriate education does not seem to occur to them. It is as though doctors and nurses feel that education is a simple matter and have no need to learn from those experienced in it. A little exposure to the experience of educators would tell medical workers that health education, especially perhaps of adults, is far from simple. There are many lessons to be learned from the disciplines of education and adult education. One of the most influential authorities in the world of adult learning is the Brazilian, Paulo Freire. His impact on health education in Third World countries has been considerable.

The contribution of Paulo Freire to education for health

Arguably, Paulo Freire has been one of the most important educationists in the world over the last two decades. His work has had an impact on thousands of educators and community development workers, including those working in health, mostly in Third World countries. Freire seems much of education in the conventional mode as part of a larger process, one of oppression: the oppression of the majority of people by a privileged minority. He sees all education as part of the process of development – or indeed underdevelopment – of people. His thinking can be seen as the application to the world of education of the 'development of underdevelopment' school of thought: those thinkers who hold that in order to make sense of the present situation with a view to improving it, we have to look at the historical economic processes of the enrichment of the few at the expense of the impoverishment of the majority. Education has played a role in this impoverishment by helping to keep people locked in a closed world. Freire is a humanist thinker and has profound religious beliefs; religion has also played a role in educating people for underdevelopment, but can be part of a positive transformation of unjust social structures. In that sense, Paulo Freire is part of another great Latin American tradition of radical Christian thinkers and activists that one would call promoters of a 'theology of liberation' (Gutierrez, 1973).

In Freire's view, education systems are major mechanisms for the perpetuation of unjust structures in society and can be themselves a form of oppression, a means of preserving inequalities. He calls for a transforming education, one which would be part of the reversal of the situation, a pedagogy of liberation. His most influential book is called *The Pedagogy of the Oppressed* (Freire, 1973). In this and his other works, Freire not only describes how oppressive much education can be, he also gives some idea of what role education can and should play in the transformation and improvement of society. He sees oppressive educational systems as working on a 'banking concept' of education, a top-down form of instruction. This is the mode of most educational systems which involve the teacher as the active agent and the learner as the passive recipient of the message. The teaching relationship, he says, is one which involves a narrating subject and listening objects. Education is suffering from 'narration sickness': 'Narration leads the students to memorise mechanically the narrated content. Worse still, it turns them into containers, into receptacles to be filled by the teacher'. Many people can recognise themselves in this simple description of top-down education, either in their memory of being educated or, more uncomfortably, perhaps, of being educators themselves: 'The more completely he (the teacher) fills the receptacles, the better a teacher he is. The more meekly the receptacles permit themselves to be filled, the better students they are' (Freire, 1973: 45).

As opposed to the 'banking concept' of education, Freire would have us consider the advantages of a problem-posing education in which learners become 'co-investigators' with the teacher. Freire's vision of society has people as subjects of transforming actions, not simply recipients or objects of such actions, having things done for them. So an appropriate and non-oppressive form of education would be one which encourages people to be active rather than passive, a participatory pedagogy (or, more awkwardly, some would speak of 'androgogy', person-centred learning, since pedagogy, strictly speaking, would refer to child-centred approaches). 'Empowerment education' would be an accurate description of Freirean pedagogy; it 'involves people in group efforts to identify their problems, to critically assess social and historical roots of problems, to envision a healthier society, and to develop strategies to overcome obstacles in achieving their goals' (Wallerstein et al, 1988: 380).

The role of the group seems of supreme importance in Freire's approach: of course, it is individuals who learn, but the support they offer to and receive from one another is significant. The 'teacher' becomes rather the facilitator of the emergence of group knowledge and confidence. Freire's original work was in literacy programmes in which he helped develop learning methods which encouraged the 'reflective participation' of learners. He speaks of reflective action on the world in order to transform it: 'Attempting to liberate the oppressed without their reflective participation in the act of liberation is to treat them as objects which must be saved from a burning building; it is to lead them into the populist pitfall and transform them into masses which can be manipulated' (Freire, 1973: 47). For some Western health workers the vocabulary is unfamiliar, but many people, despite this, find in Freire's description of education a mirror of their own experience and a hint of what education could be. Others would say that Freire presents such a powerful challenge to the establishment, is so political, that, while keeping the name of Freire, they have removed the real 'bite' of his approach; they have created a Freire without the politics, without any real challenge to the situation of oppression, a non-conflictual Freire, which they call the 'psycho-social approach' and which is not Freire at all (Kidd et al, 1979).

Empowering health education

Freire's description of 'banking education' could be an accurate description of much of what passes for health education. The health educator or health worker involved in education often sees their task as one of conveying to the less informed (if not totally ignorant) lay person some medical information necessary for the maintenance of good health. They are less likely to see their role as one of helping the patient be the 'subject of transformation' of his or her life. The Freirean vocabulary includes the word 'conscientisation', sometimes translated as 'education for critical consciousness or awareness'. It is at this point that many English-speaking health workers stop listening to Freire since they find the words unnecessarily mystifying. This is an understandable reaction, born of unfamiliarity. It is perhaps a little strange, however, for medical workers to shy away from technical or difficult terms since these are often the stock in trade of medicine. 'Conscientisation' is the educational process whereby people deepen their understanding of the limiting dimensions of their own situation and their ability to transform it.

Although Freire was not himself directly involved in health education, many health programmes have adopted his approach. Freire's pedagogy is clearly an empowering one: 'An empowering health education effort therefore involves much more than improving self-esteem, self-efficacy or other health behaviours that are independent from environmental or community change; the targets are individual, group and structural change' (Wallerstein et al, 1988: 380).

It is not difficult to see the compatibility between Freire's approach to education and the philosophy of comprehensive PHC. Primary medical care and programmes of selective PHC interventions will see no place for the kind of education promoted by Freire. Freire's philosophy, on the other hand, offers an educational framework consistent with the comprehensive PHC approach (Macdonald et al, 1991).

For Paulo Freire and those who implement his approach, the recognition of injustices in society is the starting point of a liberating education; David Werner, who has done so much in his work and in his writings to apply Freire's approach to health, accepts that following this approach of Freire makes his books explicitly political, though on the surface they may seem to be simple manuals for village health workers and their training. In PHC, one of the starting points of reflection and understanding of ill-health is the recognition of the unjust distribution of health and health resources 'between and within nations' (Alma Ata); part of the ultimate aim of this approach would be the removal of such structural obstacles to health. A PHC approach to health education would need to incorporate a dimension of equity and this will influence both the content and methods adopted.

For Freire, true education encourages the role of the learner, through participative reflection. PHC's most notable dimension and that which distinguishes it from other health-care approaches is the emphasis on participation. It is not hard to see why many programmes of PHC either explicitly invoke Freire as a guide or unconsciously mirror his approach. Freire's cautioning against 'banking' education would make health workers wary of those health education programmes which are seemingly based on assumptions of the ignorance of people about health and the need to 'fill up' this ignorance. 'Conscientisation' means becoming aware of the contradictions in one's present situation and one's ability – often together with others – to transform this situation. The PHC approach is to promote knowledge, not only of symptoms of disease, but its root causes. Again, the attraction of Freire is obvious.

Freire helps us move away from a narrow focus on the individual and individual behavioural change as the exclusive focus of health education. The individual is seen as part of a wider social economic world and elements in this world which enhance or hinder the quality of life, and therefore the health of people, are legitimate topics of an empowering health education. This is not to say that Freirean approaches to health education would pretend that there can be genuine change, including that envisaged by health education, without individual change. Empowering education has no difficulty in incorporating the perspectives of the preventive, psychological model of education; the inverse does not hold so easily. Freirean educators are not saying that there can be genuine collective change without personal learning. Freire's approach is just the opposite of the manipulation of people; for him the individual is all-important, but as a person-in-community, unique but with others and whose destiny lies in the humanising of society.

Health education: the example of the Third World

If, in terms of international perspectives of health care, we are to look for examples of health education practice which go in the direction of a PHC approach, we should be looking to the Third World, often to programmes inspired by Freirean type programmes. The West has many lessons to learn in this area. It is sad to note that many Western health education programmes and some international journals of health education seem to ignore this opportunity that the West has to learn from education initiatives in Latin America, Asia and Africa. It is as though medical technical 'superiority' blinds even progressive practitioners in the West to this possibility to learn. There is at least tacit agreement that many health education strategies 'don't work', yet all the debates about the most appropriate health education 'models' seem to turn around the West's preoccupation with the psychology of individual learning. One exception to this cultural resistance to learning from the Third World can be seen in the Swedish Health Study Circles (Strombeck, 1991). In these groups, health education is seen as a collective activity of both learning and action; its focus is not just individual behaviour but social and economic contexts as well. But there are many thinkers and practitioners of health education in the Third World whose experience of the role of groups should be taken on board by health educators everywhere. The links between 'popular' education and health in Latin America has led to exciting initiatives. Paulo Freire is part of this movement, but he has to be seen as part of a whole culture which takes seriously such notions as 'participation' and the need to build people's confidence as well as their information base. Organisations such as the Popular Education and Primary Health Care Network in Latin America and the Asian Community Health Action Network are not well enough known in the West. There is a real need for the sharing of experiences of PHC across all continents.

Chapter Nine

The Health Professional and the Macroscope

The Primary Health Care approach to health calls for a new kind of health professional and a new ideal of health work. This may sound like a bold enterprise, but it is one which cannot be shirked by promoters of PHC because the attempt to be consistent with the challenges of PHC demands nothing less. Of course, the underlying reason for the need for a new kind of health professional is that a narrow medical approach will not suffice for the health needs of populations in rich and poor countries. Moreover, once a health worker has experienced the frustrations of the constraints of health work within the framework offered by the engineering model of health care she (the feminine form will be used throughout) is already part of the move towards a new professionalism. Once the issues raised by Alma Ata and comprehensive PHC have been addressed, they are difficult for the health worker to ignore completely. It is not a tenable position to suggest that the holistic approach to health care outlined at Alma Ata is relevant only for countries of the Third World. The PHC dimensions of equity, people's participation and the need for intersectoral collaboration call into question the work of all health-care systems and those who work in them in whatever country. PHC calls for a new kind of doctor, a new kind of health worker, a new health profession.

First of all, a new understanding of health is called for. Alma Ata takes seriously the broad definition of health concerning not only the absence of disease but individual and social well-being. This definition is often attacked for being too vague and not 'scientific' enough. If science involves a reflection on what is, then we have surely shown that a concept of health mainly focused on the bio-physical inevitably misses much of what is in terms of the social and environmental causes of health and disease. Mitchell argues for concepts of health and health care which remake the connections between our ill-health and the society which 'makes us sick': 'Instead of ignoring the causes of illness, excluding them, or turning them back upon ourselves, we need health care which reinforces and strengthens our consciousness of what we are up against and our will to fight it' (Mitchell, 1984: 219).

Such an approach would certainly move away from the narrower vision of health as simply the absence of disease and pave the way for a more holistic approach. Perhaps most importantly, a health profession with such a vision of health would be led by professional impetus to adopt an integrated approach to health services. This would mean conceptualising and planning health and health care in a way which refuses to separate medicine from public health and public health from the work of groups of people struggling to create healthy conditions. Primary Health Care 'addresses the main health problems in the community, providing promotive, preventive, curative and rehabilitative services accordingly' (Alma Ata Declaration VII 2). This means that all health workers should see themselves as part of an integrated health-care system, their work would make sense as a contributory component of the whole system and could not be planned for in isolation from the whole. In this perspective, all educators of health personnel would see their task as preparing people for a place in such an integrated system, whatever the kind or level of specialisation such trainees ultimately undertook.

The new professional would be the health educator, the doctor, the nurse or other health worker who would have been trained in a basic philosophy of health and not only disease. She would be someone trained to see health care as an enterprise to be undertaken with the patient and the community and not just on their behalf and for their benefit. In other words, participation would be a normal professional concern. Grounded in a profound study of the causes of health and disease in people and in communities, such a professional would be oriented from the beginning of her training and practice to work with other sectors which she knows contribute to health. In some countries, this will mean with such sectors as agriculture and in others with social and welfare workers and in all societies it will mean a close collaboration with all aspects of the education sector. In PHC terms, intersectoral collaboration would be the norm of health professional behaviour.

The ethical perspective of such a new professional would not be restricted to a consideration of the rules of personal behaviour but would include a preoccupation with the wider dimensions of health for as many in the population as possible. In PHC terms, we are talking about the equity dimension of health care, the planning of health services dictated, not by the needs of health institutions and those who run them, but by the health needs of the majority of the population. This professional concern with the equity dimension of health and ill-health would include an understanding of the social mechanisms which impact on health; a health worker would not be able by herself to redress social imbalances, but an orientation towards 'health for all' would build in a bias for the disadvantaged.

If such a description sounds ridiculously utopian and not even worth the time for a debate, could it be because the health profession is satisfied with its existing professional image and approach? Is it unreasonable or impossible to make participation, equity and intersectoral collaboration professional preoccupations of all health workers? Is the engineering model of health care, well removed from the world of justice, people's involvement and the need to collaborate with other professionals, so well established as part of the status quo and so powerful that its underlying assumptions and philosophy are beyond questioning?

In the previous chapter, we considered education for PHC and this was understood in the sense of education of people and communities. There is another necessary area of education for PHC and that is, of course, the education of professionals. PHC can be seen as a way of looking at health care which stresses partnership between professionals and people. Individuals and communities must be educated to take more control over their health and to learn to work with health personnel. This calls for appropriate education for health of both individuals and communities. Equally, health personnel need training in the skills and attitudes required in such a partnership. This is an area which has received too little attention. But for the PHC ideals to be translated into practice, they need to be incorporated in concrete ways into the curricula of all medical training establishments. There are not, or should not be, tablets of stone on which are written the unchangeable criteria of medical training.

There are innovative practices in medical training establishments encouraged by WHO (WHO, 1991). These involve health personnel learning to work in and with communities, trained to see disease not only as biological malfunction but also as a social construct. They deserve much wider publication and discussion. Medical training establishments, sometimes the inner fortresses of the health profession, need to be involved in a vigorous examination of their purpose and product in ways suggested by the Council for International Organizations of Medical Sciences. The Council recognises the need for serious adjustment in medical training, particularly on account of 'the mismatch between training and job requirements', often coming from the demand for sophisticated medical care:

> Political pressures exerted by elitist groups have encouraged the system to over-respond to shortages, and this in turn spurred an excessive demand for medical education which is too often totally unrelated to the actual health needs of the community or what it can afford to pay for health services (Bankowski et al, 1987: 199).

Changes would involve much greater emphasis on sociological perspectives; sociology would need to move away from its present position as a poor relative to become an essential component of medical sciences and medical training.

Training for contact with individuals

A broad understanding of health and ill-health and of the consequent need for 'promotive, preventive, curative and rehabilitative services' in the spirit of Alma Ata would require considerably more emphasis on training for communication than is at present the norm for most health workers. Surely the vital part of any health-care system is the point of contact with people. All health-care systems can be seen as communication systems, involving a wide variety of communications exchange, but the most important of these exchanges, from the point of view of planning for health, is between the 'client' and the professional. Scientific knowledge and high levels of secondary and tertiary care are of extremely dubious value unless they are connected in a symbiotic way with people's needs (Paine and Siem Tjam, 1988). If, as has been argued in this book, the challenge of PHC lies in the call it makes to all health-care systems to re-orientate their services to the health needs of the populations they are supposed to serve, then the vital importance of first contact of people with the system is clear.

Abbatt (1980) illustrates well the use of 'task analysis' in the training of community health workers (CHWs), a practical application of competency-based learning curriculum development. Each important task of the CHW is analysed and divided into its component parts: the knowledge, attitudes and skills required for each activity are identified. Training proceeds on the basis of equipping CHWs accordingly. Such approaches to training are commonplace in Third World countries in PHC programmes at the grassroots level. Medical training establishments in these countries and in Western societies as well could learn a lot from this procedure for the training of all health workers who come into contact with the needs of individuals and communities. It should be noted that, beyond a mechanistic notion of training, sometimes even the description of a task analysis in health work is often a very difficult although rewarding exercise. A task analysis of a clinical procedure (such as the diagnosis and treatment of someone with acute respiratory infection) is not too difficult to delineate: the training steps follow easily. But it is more difficult to break into their component parts in the way Abbatt describes certain other essential tasks, such as the counselling of AIDS patients or their families, the animation of community discussions on communicable diseases. And if we did such a thing, how well could we say most health practitioners are actually trained for such work? What is the training given for what we call the 'therapeutic encounter'? Nurses are being trained, to some extent, to take on a partnership role with patients, to follow the 'nursing process', but given the power of the medical model, it must be recognised that it would be difficult for one cadre of health worker (and one with relatively less authority and status) to change the whole pattern of professional and popular expectations of the therapeutic encounter. Doctors, too, must be trained, not simply as medical scientists, but as person-centred health workers.

It is clear that the equity and intersectoral dimensions of the PHC approach must influence the training of health personnel of all kinds, but perhaps the most significant changes in training would come about if the participation element of PHC were to be taken seriously. If participation is seen as vital and as the intended response to be promoted in the patient wherever possible, health workers would be trained to be promoters of participation. The intended response would not be 'patient compliance' but some kind of partnership between client and professional.

Health workers are now often called upon to encourage people's participation, indeed to be the initiators of people's involvement in health. By and large they have not been trained for this task. On the contrary, the philosophy underlying most medical training at all levels has, in line with the engineering paradigm, encouraged the view that the health worker is the active agent and the patient or community the recipient of health-care activity. The WHO study group on community involvement in health (CIH) recognises this problem and calls for a commitment to training in both the theory and practice of CIH (WHO, 1991). The study group recognises that health personnel, including doctors, are not trained to encourage community involvement in health. To carry out this role calls for a change in attitude and a consequent necessary shift in the emphasis of medical training:

> CIH calls for a relationship in which the clients share power, in which they are perceived as active subjects, not primarily as objects. If this vocabulary, familiar in the world of development work and adult education, is unfamiliar to health personnel, this in itself gives some indication of the extent of the educational problem, not only as regards health personnel now in training but, just as importantly, those already trained (WHO, 1991: 20).

The recommendations of Mold and his colleagues (1991) concerning goal-oriented rather than problem-solving approaches to health care are extremely relevant here. In this perspective, the professional ethos would be the management of conditions with the patient. This would have to impact on the education and training of doctors as well as other health personnel in order to have any significant impact.

We have argued that the non-participatory mode of action which one can observe in the medical approach to a community has its origins in the basic conceptualising of health, ill-health and treatment which is part of the medical model. As medical education becomes more self-critical, it is to be hoped that the recommendations of those who suggest reform do not remain only in the realm of pious exhortation.

If the paradigm of basic clinical care moves away from the engineering model of health care towards a promotion of partnership between worker and patient, then there is some hope that this will impact on public health practice also.

Training for contact with communities

The relationship between health worker and individual patient sets the pattern for the relationship between the public health worker and the community. The move away from an engineering model of health care must involve the move towards the formation of community health personnel at all levels with appropriate knowledge, skills and attitudes, notably to promote people's participation in health matters. This calls for considerable reorientation.

In the search, however hypothetical, for a new kind of health professional and therefore, a new kind of professional model and training, we might well look to the world of community development for some guidelines.

Perhaps the first thing to say about PHC and community development (CD) is that neither should be confused with the organisation of departments which carry their name. There are 'PHC' centres in many countries, as for example, in India, which are in fact just medical centres and are not involved in any way with the three pillars of PHC. Likewise, there are departments called 'Community Development Departments' which do not necessarily represent the community development approach. It is from examples of good practice of CD that health workers should learn.

Community development represents an approach to the collective progress of communities based on a number of principles. First among these is the principle of self-reliance: instead of outside agents determining what is best for a community, the community is encouraged to decide its communal aims and to work together to achieve these. In community development, the directing force for change for improvement comes from the community itself. The approach of Primary Health Care echoes these preoccupations and the two approaches share many themes: the importance of the community; the acknowledgement that many problems in the community, including health problems, often have their roots in socio-economic conditions, etc. (Research Unit in Health and Behavioural Change, University of Edinburgh, 1989, Chapter Eight).

We have less excuse now for being naive in the matter of participation. We know it is about power and decision-making on matters which people deem to be significant for them. We also know that participation requires structures which facilitate this process. Previous promotion of people's involvement, like community development and *animation rurale* (dealt with in Chapter Five) experienced that participation involves some form of conflict, not necessarily violent, but nevertheless some redistribution of power. This was unacceptable to those who already had power and benefited from the status quo and so the vocabulary remained but only as a smokescreen for non-participatory programmes.

The reorientation of health professionals' attitudes, which must follow any real promotion of people's participation in health, can be difficult for someone trained to think in terms of health care as consisting largely of the diagnosis of a problem and the administration of a technical solution to it. A move towards what we could call the community development approach can happen as a result of the demands made on health personnel who do work in the community. There have been calls made on such health professionals to change their attitudes and working practice in order to allow more community involvement (Sathyamala, 1986). PHC calls for this shift of attitude. Alma Ata did not create this demand for a new approach, the Declaration is merely a reflection of the shift in the medical paradigm in the search for a less passive role for individuals and communities in the creation of health and the tackling of disease, sometimes because communities have demanded an enhanced role in the doctor–community partnership. At the Fourth International Congress of the World Federation of Public Health Associations in the mid 1980s, one of the main contributors in the opening plenary session called his input, 'The quest for community health: what have we learned?'. One of the principal lessons which he identified as having been learned in the last decade or two is that 'the key to health resides in the community' and the answers to communities' health problems 'are not best plucked from a passive community, but rather learned with an active and informed community'. From this, he goes on to say, it follows that what is called for is more than 'involvement': 'it is a question of empowerment, of gaining knowledge, taking actions, and utilising others' resources – a process in which people approach self-reliance for their own, and their community's health' (Joseph, 1984: 3).

In all of this we are far from the classical model of health care described in Chapter Two and much closer to the ethos and practice of community development.

The experience of PHC programmes in the Third World has shown that the management of PHC programmes requires very particular skills from the health worker. On the one hand, the PHC manager must work with and organise medical and other professional personnel who belong to bureaucratic structures and institutions. The normal difficulties of management of a health service are compounded in the case of PHC by the need to work with other sectors: education, water and sanitation etc. Moreover, there is a need to work in and with the community: people's organisations, village development committees and community health workers do not belong to the formal sector and cannot be 'managed' in the same way as workers within a bureaucracy. For this community aspect of PHC management and organisation, we again have to look to the world of community development for models of how to proceed. If we examine successful programmes of PHC, such as those described by Hilsum (1983), Arole (1975), and Heywood (1991), we can see evidence of the community development aspects of the Primary Health Care approach. Health workers have learned in such programmes to stop thinking of themselves as being the experts who have the technical solution to the health problems of communities and begin to see themselves more as collaborators with communities.

Carlaw (1988) talks of the 'shifting role of the health professional for Primary Health Care'. In his overview of examples of PHC practice in Africa he points out that community-based PHC such as called for by Alma Ata calls for a partnership between health professionals and the community, which he sees calling for 'a vast change in relationships and authority'. The practice of PHC calls for a new sort of professional. As this new professional emerges in Africa, Asia and Latin America, it is to be hoped that medical colleagues in Western societies will be forced to learn from their example. Only when this happens, and the public demand in Western society for more patient-centred approaches begins to make a change in the professional attitudes of doctors, will there perhaps begin to be a change in the way doctors and other health workers are trained.

The need for a new epidemiology

Epidemiology is said to be the main tool of public health work. At the moment, the discipline is one of medical science of a particular kind. What is needed is an 'epidemiology of health' and not just of disease. The etymology of the word, 'epidemiology' would suggest only the study of people, in this case of their health status. Western medicine's preoccupation is with disease and this has become the focus of the discipline. Moreover, it has approached its task as a science drawing mainly on the physical sciences, and this has brought about a focus not only on ill-health but on accurate measurement of disease. Most epidemiologists are happy to confine themselves to the examination and study of disease in populations. The study of health or well-being and the factors which promote it is a much less tidy matter and easily gets overlooked in what is seen to be the more important matter of analysing the hard facts of disease (Bibeau, 1981, Ho, 1982). As a result of the fact that epidemiology is generally geared to look at what is happening in terms of ill-health, rather than why it is happening, its methodologies are non-participatory. It is a study of and not with populations. Can we envisage a participatory mode for epidemiology? Certainly the PHC approach, with its emphasis on the essential role of the community in defining health and problems of ill-health would encourage efforts in this direction. It would be encouraging to see public-health doctors and other health workers involved with communities developing a new science of epidemiology which would not only take people's perceptions seriously but institute planning systems based on a participatory epidemiology.

Unfortunately, the transfer of the medical model to health work with the community or to public health often results in a scenario in which once again the health professional sees himself as the decision-maker and the community as the more passive recipient of the public health doctor's diagnosis.

Where is the role for participation in such a scenario? There does not seem to be much room for what we have seen to be significant participation, that is to say involvement in decision-making and evaluation. What participation can there be for the public and the community in 'public health' or 'community medicine'? What is their role conceived of as being – is it one of partnership with health personnel in the complex task of discovering and tackling the health needs of the community and the sources of their ill-health? Hardly. The role of the community as patient is to inform when asked and to comply when advised. In 'public health', there is not even any perceived necessity of asking the community about its needs. The 'tools' of public health as shaped by the engineering model are epidemiological initiatives, often aimed at the collection of quantifiable information in statistical form about the community: 'objective' facts, not 'inner perspectives' (Filstead, 1970), and not decisions or evaluations undertaken by the community.

Public health, in fact, rarely puts the doctor or other health worker in any position of dialogue with the community, let alone in a position which will offer the community a participatory role in decision-making. Public health has come to mean the application of scientific medicine to the community, the elaboration of epidemiological skills to provide tools for the understanding of disease and health service provision. Excellent work is done in this field. Few would challenge the important and fundamental role of epidemiology and the usefulness of its methodologies. Yet it is not too difficult to show that epidemiology has taken the form it has under the influence of Western scientific preoccupations and particularly as these have influenced clinical medicine. Epidemiology, as presently understood and practised, is clearly an application to the community of the scientific engineering model of health care spoken of in Chapter Two and suffers from the limitations of this perspective. It is concerned, overwhelmingly, with numbers and the verifiable relationship of influence between variables. The studies which it generates are often science-led, rather than public-health-led and their application to the task of improving people's health status often seems a matter of indifference to the scientists involved. As such, and in the way it has developed, it is at best a partial tool for planners of health services aimed at meeting people's health needs. Third World public health practitioners and institutions, in an understandable effort to be as 'scientific' as their Western counterparts, are often very concerned with the quantifiable to the neglect of what could be called qualitative data. As an example of this, a study of family planning in a particular African country was, typically, concerned with the number of 'acceptors', 'defaulters', the reliability of service provision in terms of contraceptives: all, it must of course be agreed, important factors and relatively easy to count. But there was little concern for what the women, or indeed the men, felt about having children, why they wanted many offspring, or any attempt to research the role which children play in the culture and economy of the country. As a tool for planning health services, epidemiology so understood must surely be limited in what it can achieve.

As should be expected in the discipline of public health coming from an allopathic model, epidemiology is disease-oriented. As we have said, it has an inbuilt orientation towards the pathological. The doctor, in a one-to-one consultancy with his patient, is not trained to draw out what is life-enhancing and health-promoting in the individual patient facing him, but rather to find out as accurately and as specifically as possible what is 'wrong' with the patient. Likewise, the public health doctor trained in the engineering model, when she is faced with the community is in an interaction in which the focus is not on finding out what is strong and health-promoting in the groups of people she is working with and their culture. Rather, the focus is inevitably on what is 'wrong'. Even the vocabulary used in this context betrays the preoccupation with pathology of the medical model: when health workers are encouraged to do a study of health in the community they are sometimes told to do a 'community diagnosis' (Bennet, 1979). This is hardly a perspective to encourage research into community practices, beliefs and structures which foster and promote health. Rather, by definition, the focus of a diagnosis is on what is pathological, the weaknesses of the community which the health professional is going to identify and put right. Burrage points out that we will generally fail to observe what we do not in the structure of our research seek to find (Burrage, 1987: 896). The Aristotelian dictum applies here: 'Whatever is received, is received according to the mode of the receiver': if health personnel are to work in partnership with the community they must have an orientation which helps them see, and seek to encourage, all the mechanisms and people in the community which promote health, as well as being equipped with an understanding of the signs and treatment of disease and the means of recording and predicting these. The disease-focused model is of considerable use in terms, for example, of acute infectious diseases. But health services are about more than these. Let us take once again the example we have used before, childbirth, surely a priority in health services anywhere in the world. Increasingly, health services in developing countries are acknowledging that the previously-held 'ideal' of every mother delivering in a health institution is at the very least impractical. There is a need to work with 'traditional birth attendants' (TBAs) and this is much promoted in PHC as we have already suggested. The epidemiological method, as a tool of public health in this matter, tends towards a collection of data (if available) on conditions such as neonatal tetanus and its causes:

> Epidemiology concerns the population aspects of ill-health. Classically, its point of departure is a disease or health problem ... The tasks of epidemiology are then to analyse its frequency and distribution in the population, to identify associated factors ... that may be important in the causation with a view to discovering the means of control, and to evaluate the impact of interventions on the rates of occurrence (Segall 1983: 33).

In the case of birth in the community this classical approach of epidemiology will provide us with useful, but limited, information, and as a methodological perspective is not of itself going to facilitate the participation of the TBAs in any programme. How does the public-health doctor, trained in public-health medicine, recognise and respect the role of TBAs whose collaboration is essential if childbirth practices worldwide are to be improved? Trained in institution-based clinical medicine, most doctors and midwives will understandably be drawn to recognise and denounce the unhygienic practices of the local practitioners. Their 'community diagnosis' will be geared to the pathological, to the diseases and the 'at-risk' behaviours of mothers and communities.

The most successful programmes of collaboration with TBAs have adopted another approach, going beyond the limitations of perspective described. By seeking out first of all what is good and strong and life-enhancing in the community's management of childbirth, often using anthropological perspectives, these successful PHC programmes have built on such valuable resources as the dedication of the TBAs to the community and the trust many community mothers have in them. Our own recent understanding of childbirth in the West, under the influence of the women's health movement, has led us to question much of what was taken for granted in 'scientific' medicine as applied to childbirth. We are now much more inclined to give value to non-supine birthing positions, to allow mothers to have more say in what position they will give birth and to encourage intimate social support for the mother in labour. All of these are the norm in the practice of many TBAs in so-called less-developed countries. Some form of community assessment might have yielded such positive aspects in traditional practice which a 'community diagnosis' might not even have seen, let alone valued. Of course, TBAs have things to learn from Western medicine, especially in terms of hygienic practice: 'clean instrument, clean hands and clean mat'. But such things are taken on board more readily. TBAs are more inclined to 'participate', when the attitude of their health-service partners is one of respect and mutual learning rather than one of putting right what is denounced as wrong and even backward. Here we have an example of the need for in-service training for health workers: participation calls for a deal of 're-learning' on the part of health personnel.

In many Third World countries the participation dimension of PHC has led to the creation of new cadres of workers. The conventional system, with a high degree of dependence on highly-paid professionals trained in curative care had made little impact on the health status of the majority of populations. In the name of PHC, village/community health workers have been trained in their thousands since the mid 1960s in preventive, educational and simple curative care. Their work has not been an unqualified success (Walt, 1990). Explanations of failures are seen to lie in their training (Jobert, 1985), low credibility, often due to lack of basic drugs (Parlato and Favin, 1982), and their selection often being unduly influenced by health professionals rather than being an expression of community choice (Matomora, 1991). These workers have had great expectations placed on them: they were to provide a health-care system at the village level which was preventive as well as curative, educational as well as rehabilitative; to be the essential implementers of PHC. For little or no rewards other than serving the community, they have been expected to promote participation, intersectoral collaboration and a more equitable health service. The irony of building this latter pillar of PHC, equity, on the work of such workers should not be missed: they themselves might be well described as oppressed, asked to do for next to nothing what the salaried medical profession has long been unable to achieve in terms of holistic care, community participation and intersectoral collaboration. India has had some form of village health worker for longer than most countries. Bose says of them, 'As for disease-preventive and health promotive work such as immunisation, waste disposal, nutrition surveillance and education, they were not trained ... to handle any of these activities without strong back-up from the Health Centre (where the doctor is based) ... and that was usually lacking' (Bose, 1983: 44).

The pattern of enormous and unrealistic expectation both from communities and professionals has been repeated in many countries. No wonder the deployment of such workers has rarely been an unqualified success and they have often been treated as 'just another pair of hands' by the medical system (Walt, 1990). It would indeed be expecting miracles to expect poorly paid and low-status health workers trained and 'managed' within this paradigm to change significantly the patterns of behaviour and expectation the model itself creates. If community-level health workers are going to succeed, they have to have back-up and genuine support from the medical profession. Where there are positive examples of village or community-level health workers, often in non governmental organisations working on a small scale, it is clear that health professionals have actively pursued a policy of partnership with these workers (Berhorst, 1975, Arole, 1975, Mukhopadhyay, 1983). Programmes of collaboration with traditional birth attendants (TBAs) have already been mentioned as some of the success stories of PHC involving deprofessionalisation: health professionals learning to share their skills with community members and also learning from them. David Werner, who has done so much to promote participation of people in PHC, says clearly that the village health worker is either 'lackey or liberator' (Werner, 1977); his handbook, *Helping Health Workers Learn* (Werner, 1982) draws on his experience of this deprofessionalisation of health care and gives practical ideas on how health personnel can empower communities in the matter of health. Werner presumes a health professional ready to 'let go'. *Helping Health Workers Learn* should be obligatory reading for all health professionals in all countries. Wolffers (1988) comes to the interesting though predictable conclusion concerning village-level workers in one of the most successful PHC programmes, that of Gonoshastya Kendra in Bangladesh, that expectations of them are too high. This programme has concluded that one can and must provide curative care in a PHC manner without putting too much on the backs of village health workers. Matomora (1991) shows us clearly that village-level workers have a chance of bringing about the aims of PHC only if the health service, and so existing medical workers, are ready to consult and work with the community and attend to its needs before appointing community-level workers to do these things. The 'failure' of some community health workers programmes should not be seen as the failure of PHC itself, but as a manifestation of the need to see PHC as a reorientation of all health professionals and not simply the handing-over of its implementation to some under-prepared and underpaid community level workers.

It is clear that for the PHC ideals to have any chance of becoming reality, something drastic has to be done about the training of health personnel. The training or re-training of health personnel may well be the most essential component of an alternative strategy of health care. Recent reflection in the nursing profession shows an awareness of the challenge of PHC to existing ways of conceiving and executing health services (Watts, 1990) and the consequences for the training of nurses. It remains to be seen whether other members of the medical profession will also rise to the challenge.

References

Abbatt, F (1980), *Teaching for better learning*, WHO, Geneva

Aarons, A and Hawes, H (1979), *Child-to-Child*, Macmillan, London

Abed, F H (1983), 'Household teaching of ORT in rural Bangladesh', *Assignment Children*, 61/62, pp. 249–265

Abel-Smith, B (1986), 'The world economic crisis. Part 1: repercussions on health', *Health Policy and Planning* 1 (3), pp. 202–213

Adult Education And Development, March 1980

Armstrong, D (1987), 'Theoretical Tensions in Biopsychosocial Medicine', *Social Science and Medicine*, 25 (11), pp. 1213–1218.

Arnstein, S R (1971), 'Eight Rungs on the Ladder of Citizen Participation', in Cahn and Posset (1971), pp. 69–91

Arole, M and Arole, R (1975), 'A comprehensive rural project in Jamkhed, India', in Newell, K W (ed.) (1975)

Ajzen, I and Fishbein, M (1980), *Understanding Attitudes and Predicting Social Behaviour*, Prentice-Hall, Englewood Cliffs

Ashton, J and Kikbusch, I (1986), *Healthy Cities – Action Strategies for Health Promotion*, WHO, Copenhagen

Ashton, J and Seymour, H (1988), *The New Public Health*, Open University Press, Milton Keynes

Bandura, A (1977a), *Social Learning Theory*, Prentice-Hall, Englewood Cliffs

Bandura, A (1977b), 'Toward a unifying theory of behavioural change', *Psychological Review* (84), pp. 191–215

Banerji, D (1984), 'Primary health care: selective or comprehensive', *World Health Forum*, vol. 5.

Banerji, D (1985), *Health and Planning Services in India*, Lok Pash, New Delhi

Banerji, D (1986), 'Hidden menace in the Universal Child Immunisation Programme', *Journal of the Indian Medical Association*, 84 (8), pp. 229–232

Bangladesh Rural Advancement Committee (BRAC) (1979), *Peasant Perceptions: Famine*, BRAC, Dhaka

Bangladesh Rural Advancement Committee (BRAC) (1980), *The Net*, BRAC, Dhaka.

Bankowski, Z and Mejia, A (1987), *Health Manpower out of Balance*, Council for International Organisations of Medical Sciences (CIOMS), Geneva

Bannerman, R H, Burton, J and Ch'en Wen-Chieh (eds) (1983), *Traditional Medicine and Health Care Coverage*, WHO, Geneva

Batten, T R (1960), *Communities and their Development*, Oxford University Press, London

Becker, M H (ed.) (1974), 'The health belief model and personal behaviour', *Health Education Monographs* 3, pp. 324–508

Berhorst, C (1975), 'The Chimaltenango development project in Guatemala' in Newell (1975), pp. 30–52

Bibeau, G (1981), 'Current and future issues for medical social scientists in less-developed countries', *Social Science and Medicine*, vol. 15A, pp. 357–370

Biddle, W W and Biddle, I J (1965), *The Community Development Process: The Rediscovery of Local Initiative*, Holt, New York

Bose, A (1983), 'The Community Health Worker Scheme: an Indian experiment', in Morley et al., (1983), pp. 38–48

Brandt, W (1980), *North–South: a Programme for Survival*, The Brandt Commission Report, Pan Books, London

Brent Community Health Council (1981), *Black People and the Health Service*, Brent Community Health Council, London

Briggs, G W and Banahan, B F (1990), 'Some pitfalls of the authoritarian doctor-patient relationships in primary care medicine', *Journal of the Mississippi State Medical Association*, vol. 31 (12), pp. 395–6

Briscoe, J (1984), 'Water supply and health in developing countries: selective primary health care revisited', *American Journal of Public Health*, 74 (9), pp. 1009–13

British Medical Journal (1990), vol. 301, 18–25 August, editorial.

Bryan, B, Dadzie, S and Scafe, S (1985), *The Heart of the Race. Black Women's Lives in Britain*, Virago, London

Bucks, R S, Williams, A, Whitfield, M J and Routh, D A (1990), 'Towards a typology of general practitioners' attitudes to general practice', *Social Science and Medicine* 30 (5), pp. 537–547

Bunton, R, Murphy, S and Bennet, P (1991), 'Theories of behavioural change and their use in health promotion: some neglected areas', *Health Education Research*, 6 (2), pp. 153–162

Burrage, H (1987), 'Epidemiology and community health: a strained connection?', *Social Science and Medicine*, 25 (8), pp. 895–903

Buttfield, I, Buttfield, B, Moorhead, R and Murrell, T G (1990), 'The role of the GP in the management of chronic disease. Diabetes as a model', *Australian Family Physician*, 19 (8), pp. 1187–9, 1193–6, 1199

Cahn, E S and Posset, B A (1971), *Citizen Participation: Effecting Community Change*, Praeger, New York

Caplan, A, Englehardt, H T and McCartney, J J (1981), *Concepts of Health and Disease. Interdisciplinary Perspectives*, Addison-Wesley, Reading, Mass.

Carlaw, R W and Ward, W B (eds) (1988), *Primary Health Care: The African Experience*, Third Party Publishing Company, Oakland, California

Chambers, R (1983), *Rural Development: Putting the Last First*, Longman, Harlow

Chen, L C (1988), 'Ten years after Alma Ata: balancing different primary health care strategies', *Tropical and Geographical Medicine* 40 (3), pp. 522–529

Chowdhury, A M R (1990), 'Empowerment through health education: the approach of an NGO in Bangladesh', in Streefland et al. (eds) (1990), pp. 113–120

CINI (Child in Need Institute, West Bengal), (1988), personal communication, March 14

Cisse, B M (1964), 'Animation rurale, Senegal's road to development', *Community Development Bulletin*, vol. 15, no. 2

Cohen, J M and Uphoff, N T (1977), *Rural Development Participation: Concepts and Measures for Project Design, Implementation and Evaluation*, Cornell University Rural Development Committee, Ithaca

Cohen, J M, Uphoff, N T and Goldsmith, A A (1979), *Feasibility and Application of Rural Development Participation: A State-of-the-Art Paper*, Cornell University Rural Development Committee, Ithaca

Cohen, J M and Uphoff, N T (1980), 'Participation's place in rural development: seeking clarity through specificity', *World Development* 8, pp. 213–235

Coleman, V (1988), *The Health Scandal*, Sidgwick and Jackson, London

Crawford, R (1977), 'You are dangerous to your health: the ideology and politics of victim-blaming', *International Journal of Health Services*, 7, pp. 663–80

Crawford, R (1980), 'Healthism and the medicalisation of everyday life', *International Journal of Health Services*, 10, pp. 365–388

Descartes, R ([1637, 1641], 1968), *Discourses on Method and the Meditations*, translation by F E Sutcliffe, Penguin, London

DHSS (Department of Health and Social Security) (1980), *Inequalities in Health*, report of a research working group, HMSO, London

Douglas, M (ed.) (1971), *Understanding Everyday Life. Toward The Reconstruction of Sociological Knowledge*, Routledge and Kegan Paul, London

Doyal, L (1979), *The Political Economy of Health*, Pluto Press, London

Dubos, R (1959), *Mirage of Health*, Harper and Row, New York

Economist (1986), 'Primary Health care is not curing Africa's ills', May 31, pp. 97–100

Ehrenreich, B and English, D (1978), *For Her Own Good*, Anchor Press, New York

Eng, E, Briscoe, J and Cunningham, A (1990), 'Participation effect from water projects on EPI', *Social Science and Medicine*, 30 (12), pp. 1349–58

Engel, G L (1976), 'The need for a new medical model: a challenge for bio-medicine', *Science*, 196, no. 4286

Evans, R G and Stoddardt, G L (1990), 'Producing health, consuming health care', *Social Science and Medicine*, vol. 31, no. 12

FAO (1980), *Ideas and Action* 134 (2)

Fabricant, S J and Hirschorn, N (1987), 'Deranged distribution, perverse prescription, unprotected use: the irrationality of pharmaceuticals in the developing world', *Health Policy and Planning*, 2 (3), pp. 204–213

Farrant, W (1989), 'Health promotion and community health movement: experiences from the UK', paper presented at the International Symposium on Community Participation and Empowerment Strategies in Health Promotion, Biefeld University, Germany, June

Fassin, D (1991), 'Les origines sociales des inégalites de santé en Ecuador', *Cahiers Santé* 1 (1), pp. 25–32

Filstead, W J (1970), *Qualitative Methodology* Markham, Chicago

Fitzroy, H, Briend, A and Faveau, V (1990), 'Child survival: should the strategy be redesigned? Experience from Bangladesh, *Health Policy and Planning*, 5 (3), pp. 1–9

Franco-Agudelo, S (1983), 'The Rockefeller Foundation's antimalarial programme in Latin America: donating or dominating?', *International Journal of Health Services*, 13 (1)

Frank, A G (1967), *Capitalism and Underdevelopment in Latin America*, Monthly Review Press, New York

Fraser, W and Meli, J (1990), 'Maternal health services – the developing world', *Canadian Journal of Public Health*, 81 (6), pp. 436–8

Freire, P (1973), *Pedagogy of the Oppressed*, Penguin, London

Government of Zambia (1981), *Health by the People*, Ministry of Health, Lusaka

Gilson, L (1988), 'Health sector financing: a response to Oscar Gish', *Health Policy and Planning*, 3 (1), pp. 77–79

Gilson, L (1989), 'What is the future for equity within health policy?', *Health Policy and Planning*, 4 (4), pp. 323–327

Graham, H (1986), 'Women smoking and family health', paper presented at the British Sociological Association Medical Sociology Group Conference, September, York

Green, L W, Kreuter M W, Deeds, S G and Partridge, K B (1980), *Health Education Planning: A Diagnostic Approach*, Mayfield Publishing, Palo Alto

Grodos, D and de Bethune, X (1988), 'Les interventions sanitaires sélectives: un piège pour les politiques de santé du Tiers Monde', *Social Science and Medicine*, 26 (9), pp. 879–889

Gutierrez, G (1973), *A Theology of Liberation*, Orbis Books, Marylknoll

Hall, B L (1978), *Tanzania's Health Campaign*, Clearing House on Development Communication, Washington

Harpham, T, Lusty, T and Vaughan, P (eds) (1988), *In the Shadow of the City. Community Health and the Urban Poor*, Oxford University Press, Oxford

Heywood, A (1991), *Primary Health Care in the Atacora, Benin. Successes and Failures*, Royal Tropical Institute, Amsterdam

Hilsum, L (1983), 'Nutritional education and social change: a women's movement in the Dominican Republic', in Morley, D et al (eds), pp. 114–132

Holdcroft, L E (1978), *The Rise and Fall of Community Development in Developing Countries, 1950–1965*, MSU Rural Development Papers, Michigan State University, Paper no. 2

Hongelian, Y, Yiheng, M, Xiuchen, Q, Hualin, Z, Qibin, L, Jihui, G and Clayton, S, 'A Multisectoral Approach to Primary Health Care in Fujian, China', *Health Education Quarterly*, 18 (1), pp. 17–27

Hope, A and Timmel, S (1984), *Training for Transformation. A Handbook for Community Workers*, Mambo Press, Gweru

Horn, J S (1971), *Away with All Pests*, Monthly Review Press, New York

Huang, S (1988), 'Transforming China's collective health care system: a village study', *Social Science and Medicine*, 27 (9), pp. 879–888

Illich, I (1975), *Medical Nemesis*, Caldar and Boyars, London

Janz, K N and Becker, M H (1984), 'The health belief model: a decade later', *Health Education Quarterly* 11 (1), pp. 1–47

Job-Spira, N, Spencer, B, Moatti, J P, Bouvet, E (eds) (1990), *Santé publique et maladies à transmission sexuelles*, John Libbey, Paris

International Labour Office (ILO) (1978), *The Basic Needs Approach to Development*, ILO, Geneva

Jobert, B (1985), 'Populism and health policy: the case of Community Health Volunteers in India', *Social Science and Medicine*, 20 (1), pp. 1–25

Johnston, R (in print), 'Learning to Work With People. An Experience of Health Workers in Ireland' in Jones, J and Macdonald, J, special issue of *Community Development Journal* on community development and health. (Scheduled 1993)

Jones, J (1983), *Community Development and Health Issues. A Review of Existing Theory and Practice*, Community Projects Foundation, Edinburgh

Jones, J (1990), 'Community Development and the Health Service', Winter School on Community Development and Health, Paper A3, Health Education Authority/Open University

Joseph, S C (1984), 'Quest for community health: What lessons have we learned?', opening plenary session, Fourth International Congress of Public Health Associations, in *Public Health Reviews*, vol. 12, pp. 3–4

Justice, J (1987), 'The bureaucratic context of international health', *Social Science and Medicine*, 25 (12), pp. 1307–1320

Kanji, N (1989), 'Charging for drugs in Africa: UNICEF's "Bamako Initiative"', *Health Policy and Planning*, 4 (1), pp. 110–120

Kasongo Project Team (1981), 'Influence of measles vaccination on survival patterns of 7–35 months-old children in Kasongo, Zaire', *Lancet*, 4 April, pp. 764–768

Keith, Sir A (1919), *The Engines of the Human Body*, Williams and Norgate, London

Kennedy, I (1983), *The Unmasking of Medicine*, Allen and Unwin, London

Khan, A H (1985), *Rural Development in Pakistan*, Vanguard Books, Lahore

Kidd, R and Kumar, K (1979), 'Co-opting Freire: a critical analysis of pseudo-Freirean adult education', mimeo, Participatory Research Group, Toronto

Kindervatter, S (1979), *Nonformal Education as an Empowering Process*, Centre for International Education, Amherst

Klouda, A (1983), 'Prevention is more costly than cure: health problems for Tanzania, 1971–81', in Morley et al. (1983), pp. 49–63

Korten, D C (1980), 'Community organization and rural development: a learning process approach', *Public Administration Review*, Sept/Oct, pp. 480–511

Kume, J B (1980), 'Some factors influencing the mortality of under-fives in a rural area of Kenya: a multivariate analysis', *Journal of Tropical Pediatrics*, 26 (June)

Laing, R (1986), *Health and Health Services For Plantation Workers*, EPC Publication no. 10, London School of Hygiene and Tropical Medicine, London

Lankester, T E (1991), 'Primary health care: delivery or participation?', Editorial, *Tropical Doctor* 21 (1), pp. 1–2

Larrain, J (1989), *Theories of Development: Capitalism, Colonialism and Dependency*, Polity Press, Cambridge

Liberian Health Worker, personal communication, May 1987

Link (Newsletter of the Asian Community Health Action Network) (1990), 9 (2)

Lipton, M and de Kadt, E (1988), *Agriculture-Health Linkages*, WHO Offset Publications no. 104, Geneva

MacCormack, C P (1989), 'Technology and women's health in developing countries', *International Journal of Health Services*, 19 (4), pp. 681–692

Macdonald, J J (1981), *The Theory and Practice of Integrated Rural Development*, Manchester University

Monographs no. 19, Department of Education, Manchester

Macdonald, J J (1982), 'The primary health care worker as educator', Occasional Paper, no. 4, Department of Adult and Higher Education, Manchester University, Manchester

Macdonald, J J (1986), *Participatory Evaluation and Planning as an Essential Component of Community Development*, Ph.D. thesis, Manchester University, Manchester

Macdonald, J J (1987), Class record notes, PHC courses, Manchester University, Manchester

Macdonald, J J (1988), 'Collaboration for health: easy to understand, difficult to achieve', *Africa Health*, Special Supplement, November, pp. 1–4

Macdonald, J J (1990), 'La prévention des MST: une approche par le concept de soins de santé primaires', in Job-Spira et al (1990)

Maglacas, A M (1984), 'Health for all: a framework for action', *Philippine Journal of Nursing* 54 (3), pp. 78–98

Maguire, P (1984), 'Communication skills in primary care', in Steptoe and Mathews (1984), pp. 153–173

Mahler, H (1975), 'Health – a demystification of medical technology', *The Lancet*, 1 November, pp. 829–833

Marshall, T and Yanz, L (1988), *Perspectives and Practice: Health and Popular Education in Latin America*, International Council for Adult Education, Toronto

Martin, P (1983), *Community Participation in Primary Health Care*, American Public Health Association, *Primary Health Care Issues*, Series 1 (5), Washington

Martin, C J, Platt, S D and Hunt, S M (1987), *Housing Conditions and Ill-health*, BMJ, 294, pp. 1125–1127

Matomora, M K (1989), 'Mass-produced village health workers and the promise of primary health care', *Social Science and Medicine*, 28 (10), pp. 1081–1084

McAnany, E G (1980), *Communications in the Rural Third World*, Praeger, New York

McCormack, C, personal communication, 3 August, 1991

McEvers, N (1980), 'Health and the assault on poverty in low-income countries', *Social Science and Medicine*, vol. 14C, pp. 41–57

McKeown, T (1976), *The Role of Medicine: Dream, Mirage or Nemesis?*, Nuffield Provincial Hospitals Trust, London

McKinley, J B (1979), 'A case for refocusing upstream: the political economy of illness', in Jaco, E G (ed.) (1979), *Patients, Physicians and Illness*, Free Press, New York

McWhinney, I R (1983), 'Changing models: the impact of Kuhn's theory on medicine', *Family Practice* 1,1

Medawar, C and Freese, B (1982), *Drug Diplomacy*, Social Audit, London

Medawar, C (1984), *Drugs and World Health*, Social Audit, London

Mehmet, O (1978), *Economic Planning and Social Justice in Developing Societies*, Croom Helm, London

Mercado, R D (1990), 'Report: the 32nd SEAMO-TROPMED Regional Seminar: Primary Health Care as a participative approach in the improvement of the quality of life' *South-East Asian Journal of Tropical Medicine and Public Health*, 21 (3), pp. 334–346

Mitchell, J (1984), *What Is To Be Done About Illness and Health?*, Penguin, Harmondsworth

Mold, J W, Blake, G H, Becker, L A (1991), 'Goal-oriented medical care', *Family Medicine* 23 (1), pp. 46–51

Moran, G (1986), 'Radical health promotion: a role for Local Authorities?', in Rodmell and Watt (1986), pp. 121–138

Morley, D, Rhode, J and Williams, G (eds) (1983), *Practising Health for All*, Oxford University Press, Oxford

Mosley, W H (1988), 'Is there a middle way? Categorical programs for PHC', *Social Science and Medicine*, 26 (9), pp. 907–908

Moulton, J M (1977), *Animation Rurale: Education for Rural Development*, University of Massachusetts, Amherst

Mukhopadhyay, M (1983), 'Human development through primary health care: case studies from India', in Morley et al (1983)

Naidoo, J (1986), 'Limits to individualism', in Rodmell and Watt (1986), pp. 17–37

Navarro, V (1984), 'A critique of the ideological and political positions of the Willy Brandt Report and the WHO Alma-Ata Declaration', *Social Science and Medicine* 18, pp. 467–474

Navarro, V (1986), *Crisis, Health and Medicine*, Tavistock, London

Newell, K W (ed.) (1975), *Health by the People*, WHO, Geneva

Newell, K W (1988), 'Selective Primary Health Care: the counter revolution', *Social Science and Medicine* 26 (9), pp. 903–906

Newton, J (1988), *Preventing Mental Illness* Routledge, London

Nissinen, A, Tuomilehto, J and Puska, P (1988), 'From pilot project to national implementation: experiences from the North Karelia Project', *Scandanavian Journal of Primary Health Care*, 1, Supplement, pp. 49–56

O'Sullivan, J (1980), 'Guatemala: marginality and information in rural development in the Western Highlands' in McAnany (1980), pp. 71–106

O'Sullivan-Ryan, J and Kaplun, M (undated), *Communication Methods to Promote Grassroots Participation*, Communication and Society no. 6, Unesco, Paris

Paine, L H W and Siem Tjam, F (1988), *Hospitals and the Health Care Revolution*, WHO, Geneva

Parlato, M B and Favin, M N (1982), *Primary Health Care: Progress and Problems. An Analysis of 52 AID-Assisted Projects*, American Public Health Association, Washington

Pelletier, K R (1979), *Holistic Medicine. From Stress to Optimum Health*, Dele Publishing Company, New York

Popular Education and Primary Health Care Network (1989), *Health and Popular Education*, Newsletter no. 10, April

Prentice-Dunn, S and Rogers, R W (1986), 'Protection Motivation Theory and preventive health: beyond the health belief model', *Health Education Research* 1 (3), pp. 153–161

Puffer, R R and Serrano, C V (1973), *Patterns of Mortality in Childhood*, PAHO, Scientific Publications, in Sanders (1985)

Rifkin, S B and Walt, G (1986), 'Why health improves: defining the issues concerning "comprehensive primary health care" and "selective primary health care"', *Social Science and Medicine* 23 (6), pp. 559–566

Rodmell, S and Watt, A (1986), *The Politics of Health Education*, RKP, London

Rodney, W (1972), *How Europe Underdeveloped Africa*, Bogle L'Ouverture, London

Rogers, E M (1969), *Modernization Among Peasants*, Rinehart and Winston, New York

Rosenstock, I M, Strecher, V J and Becker, M H (1988), 'Social learning theory and the health belief model', *Health Education Quarterly* 15 (2), pp. 175–183

Rostow, W W (1960), *The Stages of Economic Growth*, Cambridge University Press, London

RUHBC (Research Unit in Health and Behavioural Change, University of Edinburgh) (1989), *Changing The Public Health*, John Wiley, Chichester

Ryan, W (1976), *Blaming the Victim*, Vintage Press, New York

Sabatier, R C (1989), 'AIDS education: evolving approaches', *Canadian Journal of Public Health*, 80, Supplement 1, pp. S9–S11

Sanders, D (1985), *The Struggle For Health*, Macmillan, London

Sathyamala, C, Sundharam, N and Bhanot, N (1986), *Taking Sides: The Choices Before the Health Worker*, Anitra, Madras

Savage King, F (1991), personal communication

Segall, M (1983), 'The politics of primary health care', *IDS Bulletin* 14 (4) (*Health, Society and Politics*), pp. 27–37

Sidel, R and Sidel, V W (1982), *The Health of China*, Beacon Press, Boston

Steptoe, A and Mathews, A (eds) (1984), *Health Care and Human Behaviour*, Academic Press, London

Streefland, P and Chabot, J (eds) (1990), *Implementing Primary Health Care. Experiences since Alma Ata,* Royal Tropical Institute, Amsterdam

Strombeck, R (1991), 'The Swedish study circle – possibilities for application to health education in the United States', *Health Education Research* 6 (1), pp. 7–17

Tarimo, E and Creese, A (eds) (1990), *Achieving Health For All by the Year 2000. Midway Reports of Country Experiences*, WHO, Geneva

Tones, K, Tilford, S and Robinson, Y K (1990), *Health Education. Effectiveness and Efficiency*, Chapman and Hall, London

Townsend, P and Davidson, N (eds) (1982), *Inequalities in Health*, Pelican, London

Townsend, P, Davidson, N and Whitehead, M (1990), *Inequalities in Health*, Penguin, London

Traitler, R (1974), *People's Participation in Development. A Reflection on the Debate*, CCPPD, World Council of Churches (Document 4), Geneva

UNDP (United Nations Development Programme) (1990), *Human Development Report*, 1990, Oxford University Press, Oxford

UNDP (United Nations Development Programme) (1992), *Human Development Report*, 1992, Oxford University Press, Oxford

UNICEF (1984), *The State of the World's Children*, Oxford University Press/UNICEF, Oxford

UNICEF (1991), *The State of the World's Children*, Oxford University Press/UNICEF, Oxford

UNRISD (United Nations Research Institute for Social Development), *Enquiry into Participation – A Research Approach* (edited by A Pearse and M Stiefel), UNRISD, Geneva

Wallerstein, N and Bernstein, E (1988), 'Empowerment education: Freire's ideas adapted to health education', *Health Education Quarterly*, 15 (4), pp. 379–394

Walsh, J A and Warren, K S (1979), 'Selective primary health care: an interim strategy for disease control in developing countries', *Social Science and Medicine*, 14C, pp. 145–163, reprinted from *New England Journal of Medicine*, vol. 301

Walt, G (ed.) (1990), *Community Health Workers in National Programmes. Just Another Pair of Hands?*, Open University Press, Milton Keynes

Walton, H J (1983), 'The place of primary health care in medical education in the UK: a survey', *Medical Education*, 17, pp. 141–147

Walton, H J (1985), 'Primary health care in European medical education: a survey' *Medical Education*, 19, pp. 167–188

Warren, K S (1988), 'The evolution of selective primary health care', *Social Science and Medicine* 26 (9), pp. 891–898

Werner, D (1977), 'The village health worker, lackey or liberator?', mimeo, paper presented at the International Hospital Federation Congress, Tokyo

Werner, D (1978), *Where There Is No Doctor*, (revised edition), The Hesperian Foundation, Palo Alto

Werner, D (1982), *Helping Health Workers Learn*, Hesperian Foundation, Palo Alto

Werner, D (1987), *Disabled Village Children*, Hesperian Foundation, Palo Alto

Werner, D (1988), 'Empowerment and health', *Contact*, no. 102, World Council of Churches

World Bank (1990), *World Development Report*, World Bank, Washington

Whitehead, M (1990), 'The health divide', in Townsend, Davidson and Whitehead, 1990

Whitehead, M (1991), 'The concepts and principles of equity and health', *Health Promotion International*, 6 (3), pp. 217–228

WHO/UNICEF (1978), *Primary Health Care: The Alma Ata Conference*, WHO, Geneva

WHO (1981), *Community Control of Cardiovascular Diseases. The North Karelia Project*, WHO, Copenhagen

WHO (1983), *New Approaches to Health Education in Primary Health Care*, Technical Report Series, 690, WHO, Geneva

WHO (1985), *Targets for Health for All*, WHO, Copenhagen

WHO (1986a), *Intersectoral Action for Health*, WHO, Geneva

WHO (1986b), 'Report of the Working Group on the Concept and Principles of Health Promotion' (1984), *Health Promotion*, 1 (1), pp. 73–76

WHO (1986c), *Ottawa Charter for Health Promotion. An International Conference on Health Promotion, 17–26 November 1986*, WHO, Copenhagen

WHO (1987), *Health Promotion: Concepts and Principles in Action. A Policy Framework*, WHO, Copenhagen

WHO (1988), *From Alma Ata to the Year 2000. Reflections at the Midpoint*, WHO, Geneva

WHO (1991), *Community Involvement in Health Development: Challenging Health Services*, Technical Report Series, 809, WHO, Geneva

Wilkinson, R (1991), 'Inequality is bad for your health', *The Guardian*, Wednesday, 12 June, p. 21

Wilkinson, R (1992), 'Income distribution and life expectancy', *British Medical Journal*, 304, pp. 165–168

Wisner, B (1988), *Power and Need in Africa*, Earthscan, London

Wolffers, I (1988), 'Limitations of the primary health model. A case study from Bangladesh', *Tropical and Geographical Medicine* 40 (1), pp. 45–53

World Bank (1990), World Development Report, World Bank, Washington

Yacoob, M, Brieger, W and Watts, S (1989), 'Primary health care: why has water been neglected?', *Health Policy and Planning* 4 (4), pp. 328–333

Yahya, S and Roesin, R (1990), 'Indonesia: implementation of the health-for-all strategy', in Tarimo and Creese (eds) (1990), pp. 133–150

Zimmerman, R S and Connor, C (1989), 'Health promotion in context: the effect of significant others on health behaviour change', *Health Education Quarterly*, 161, pp. 57–75

Zschock, D K (1989), 'Health sector disparities in Peru', *Bulletin of PAHO*, 22 (3), pp. 323–336

Index